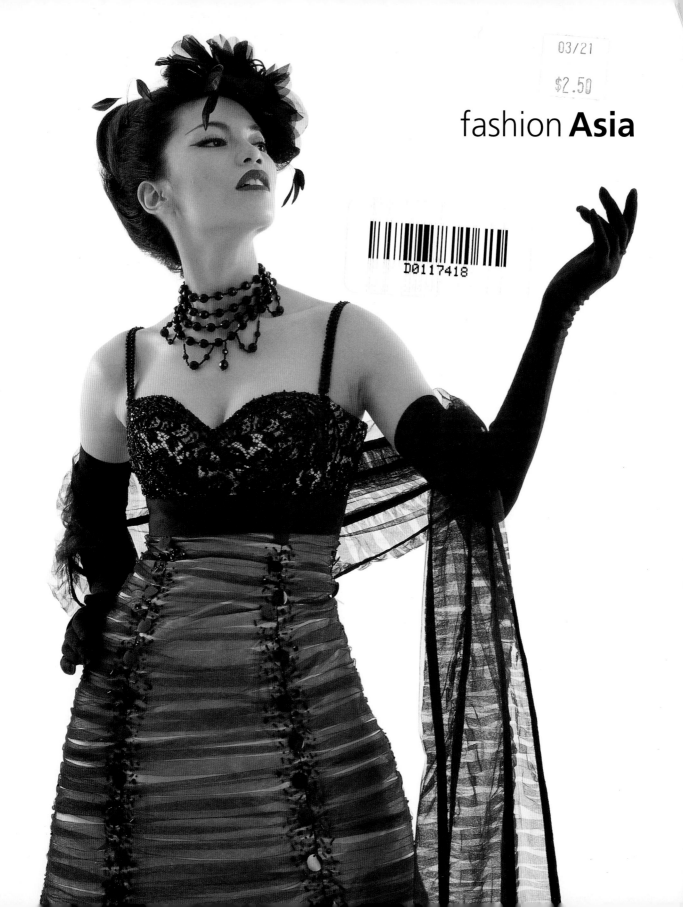

03/21

$2.50

fashion **Asia**

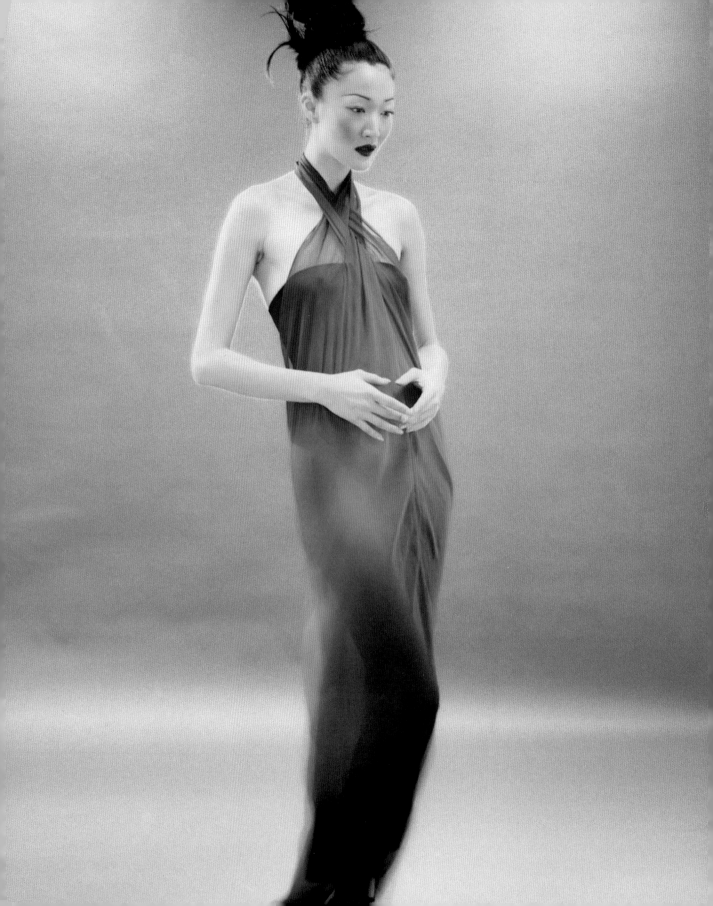

fashion **Asia**

Douglas Bullis

with 242 colour illustrations

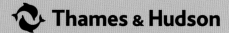
Thames & Hudson

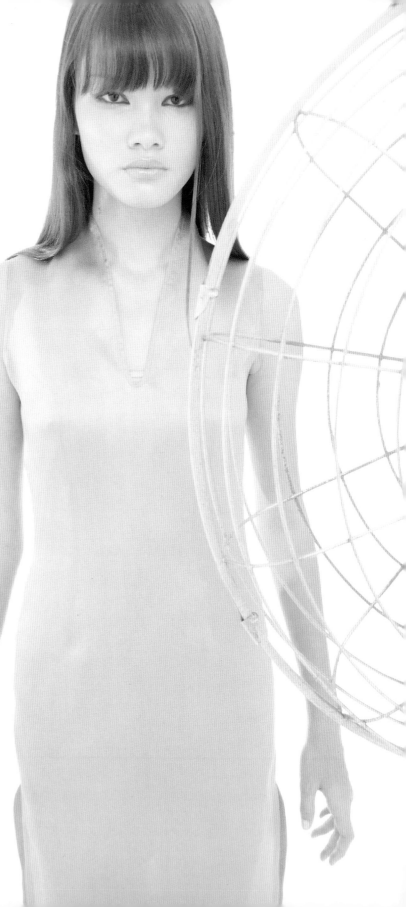

To Diane
For whose inner beauty books as
this shall always be written.

First published in the United Kingdom in 2000
by Thames & Hudson Ltd, 181A High Holborn,
London WC1V 7QX

www.thamesandhudson.com

British Library Cataloguing-in-Publication Data
A catalogue record for this book is available from
the British Library

Design by Broadbase

ISBN 0-500-28238-2

Printed and bound in Hong Kong by Dai Nippon

Half-title page: Design by Sebastian Gunawan
Frontispiece: Design by Celia Loe
Right: Design by Song & Kelly

Contents

Preface

Asia is fortunate in not having an inbred fashion press that influences too strongly what fashion designers think and who they will become. Most designers are delighted about this. It gives them freedom in an area where most designers are constrained – fearing what the press will say and inevitably responding to that fear by second-guessing.

You and their clients are the chief beneficiaries of this. We felt we should bring to you the life of Asian fashion in the purest form we could. Indeed, a preoccupation with purity is one of the most striking features of fashion in many parts of Asia. What looks like minimalism is not a mere paring down of unnecessities but rather the building up of a more serene self. What looks like fussy ornamentalism is really homage to a highly idealized past. From Taoism to Buddhism, from Sufi to Yogacara, the ideal is a relinquishment of the self, resulting in an inarticulable calm.

The other notable feature of Asian fashion is its devotion to detail. Devotion has two meanings here. The first is attentiveness. The second is the conveyance of spiritual messages by enmeshing them into decoration. Hence I have relied strongly on quick, impressionistic notes scribbled as the designers spoke into a tape recorder, worked with their models backstage, interrupted an interview to give instructions, or dawdled over dinner at the end of a hard day. Many other thoughts were jotted down without reflection during fashion shows, with no preconceptions getting in the way.

In re-creating these designers' worlds, I have sometimes strayed from the conventional ideas of fashion prose. Indeed, I have sought to examine Asian fashion as an art form, rather than as a commercial vehicle. Similarly, too, Asian designers themselves stray from the conventions of fashion vocabulary and merchandizing.

I have adopted the most non-judgmental sequence I could think of – listing the designers alphabetically – so that you, the readers, can draw your own conclusions. To give some sense of the regional diversity in design thinking, the chapters journey northwards, starting with the southern tier of designers in Indonesia and finishing with China.

Most importantly, I have tried as far as possible to avoid being the middle-man between you and the designers. The brief summaries are my own observations, but, in the personal statements, I remove the author's hand entirely and take you directly into the minds of these artists. I asked them to imagine themselves sitting with you over a cup of coffee, describing to you their lives, ambitions, failures, ideas, impulses, visions, joys. I wanted you to experience first-hand what goes through their minds when they first lay eyes on a perfect piece of cloth; what goes through their hearts when they see a perfect curve; what it is like to be in their nervous system as they walk down the runway to a thundering burst of applause.

Unfortunately, there was not enough space to include all of the designers I would have liked to in this book. Inevitably, personal tastes and prefer-ences played an important role, but they were not the only consideration. The Western custom of documenting one's career with publication-quality transparencies is regrettably still to take hold in Asia. As a result, certain designers who were unable to provide photographs of their work were left out to make space for the wealth of talented designers who could. Let's hope that they address this issue and are able to do so in the future. After all, good pictures cost much less than a catwalk show and last a lot longer.

The result, I hope, is a living portrait of a little-known – and certainly under-appreciated – fashion corner of the world. Given Asia's truly immense garment ancestry and diversity, it is surprising that so few have been watching closely their fashion designers of today. They are certainly worth it.

Douglas Bullis
Mirissa, Sri Lanka

Introduction

Design by Song & Kelly

Asia's Culture Couture

A timeless garment needs but two qualities: roots and wings. Yet despite such simple and elegant constants, fashion has evolved into a complex and fugitive art. It is difficult to pin down. It grasps at the moment. Tomorrow is another day, another mood, another colour, another shape.

Despite its fluttering from flower to flower, fashion is an art of form and permanence just like any other. It relies on an underlying structure in the same way that architecture does – 'elevation' may be called 'silhouette', but it still defines shape at a distance. As with sculpture, form is created by adding to or removing from. A garment responds to strokes and palette the same way a canvas does. In a painting, broad brushwork establishes theme and mood; fine brushwork embroiders a memorable image. With fashion, the broad brush is fabric and colour; the details are cut, styling and accessories.

But unlike art destined for the wall or the pedestal, fashion has a quality it shares only with dance: it changes as the body moves. Fashion's fleetingness is dictated by surroundings – wind, movement, light, time of day, the form and spirit of the wearer.

This book is about Asian fashion's form and spirit as it is expressed in the different ideals of Indonesia, Singapore, Malaysia, Thailand, the Philippines, Taiwan, Hong Kong and China. There should be no sense of hierarchy imputed into this order; the intention is to juxtapose as vividly as possible design traditions which are quite at variance with each other.

Silk Sea

In the West, the garment's history is simple: clothing became costume and costume became couture. Couture – an arrangement of a few yards of fabric which can be recognized as the work of a specific designer – is an ephemeral art tinkering with taste and time. It attempts to harness theatre's willing suspension of disbelief to social attitudes based mainly on envy. Hence seasonal lines, the catwalk's relationship with journalism, opening nights at the opera, breathless tabloid reportage, the idea that the garment can give life to the self, and the mutual covenant that fashion and social standing are one and the same.

Three decades ago, that conception began to change with the work of Issey Miyake, Rei Kawakubo and Yohji Yamamoto. Their designs introduced the idea that fashion is a contemplation of becoming, akin to that of the Noh actor who must not enter the stage without first looking at himself, alone and in full costume, in a mirror, transforming himself into the character he is about to be. The idea being that it is the psyche that gives life to the self.

Yet be it food or interiors or philosophy, Japan is a world apart, even from its neighbours. The rest of Asia's designers have an entirely different view of things. To them the garment is not a transformation of the psyche, it is a lineage that began thousands of years ago and will continue thousands of years hence. It is the breath of the artist inhaling the presence of everything that has passed and exhaling everything to come. Fashion garbs but a daub of the self on the canvas of a

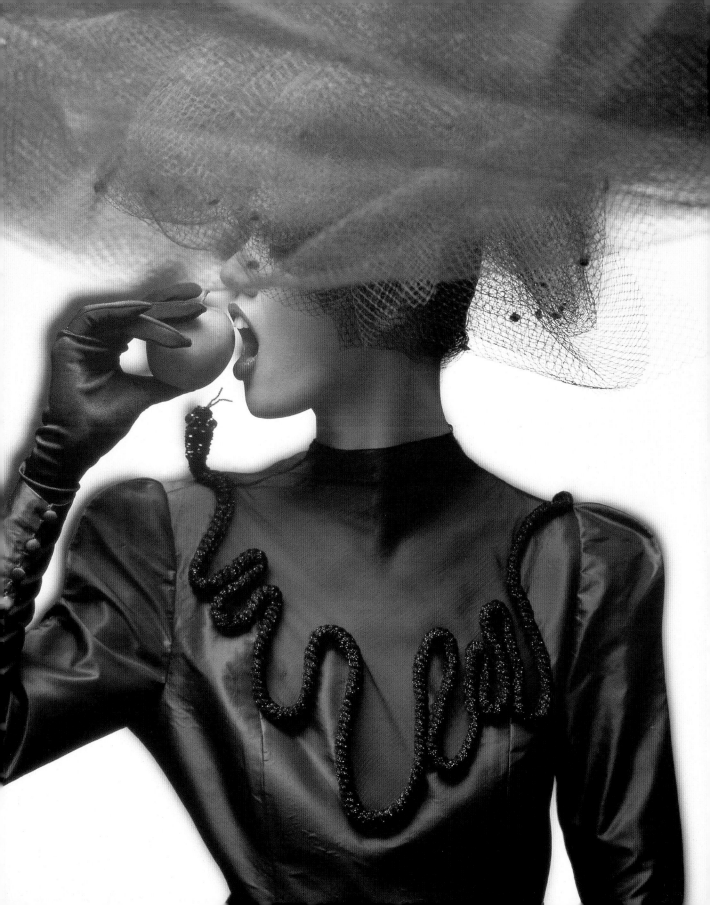

vast unity. The Asian garment expresses both timelessness and the immediacy of the present. Like the seasonless days with their unvarying hours of sun, the garment too is seasonless.

No one knows where this mentality came from. Perhaps it was from a spirit of place which juxtaposes sprawling overcrowded cities with vast uncharted jungles. Perhaps it comes from a history not of the Silk Road but of the Silk Sea. It is a view expressed in the writings of al-Ghazzali, who saw the ordinary as the mirror of the extraordinary. The Indian Theory of the Senses (*Rasa*) of 1,300 years ago speaks of the emotion of stepping out of the chiaroscuro of half-existing things into the eloquent hues of timelessness. Rabindranath Tagore says that if you can't see the soul, you see nothing. Malaysia's Syed Ahmad Jamal speaks of the eye within the soul that turns an object into an identity. The Islamic theory of the Fruit of Discourse (*'Ilm-al-Balagha*) says that ineffable truth can be glimpsed behind the masks of eloquence. And, according to the *Tao Te Ching:*

Shape truth into a vessel.
Profit comes from what is there,
Usefulness from what is not.

These notions pervade many Asian ideas about beauty. They are a sigh over centuries breathing soul into form.

In many of the statements made by the designers in this book, the words for 'garment' are used to mean 'wearer'. As they articulate their sense of tradition, it becomes clear that they are not merely fashion designers, but a continuum of artists speaking through the vocal cords of the names in this book.

Whereas the Western designer believes, 'My taste is the passing season. I give life to all that shimmers. In my wake is oblivion', the Indonesian designer Ghea Panggabean says, 'I am at one with the earliest and most recent garments of mankind.'

Old Wine in New Bottles

Asians from Beijing to Bali have constantly had to reinvent their aesthetic attitudes. For two thousand years their social equilibrium has been relentlessly overrun by economic and religious change: the multitudes of Mongols spewing out of the starvation of the Steppes; the influx of Hindu traders from the tenth to fourteenth centuries; coast-hugging Islam bearing Qur'an but no sword; colonial mercantilism and Christianity making the sixteenth to nineteenth centuries a misery; massive Chinese and Indian migrations in the nineteenth; and export-driven industrialism in the twentieth. Although such events brought retrenchment behind the secure walls of traditional social covenants and religious values, they also created the urge to try out new aesthetic ideas.

You see it evolving in the art-soul of Asia. Interiors, architecture, flower arrangements, web pages, magazine layouts, type fonts, photographs, the sense that irreducibility is as necessary today as intricate embroidery was a century ago. The art-soul is in the air, you can't help but breathe it. Whether it is Singapore's vividly coloured but minimalist sculptured look, the totemistic theatrical productions masquerading as catwalk shows in Hong Kong, the Philippine wedding as the

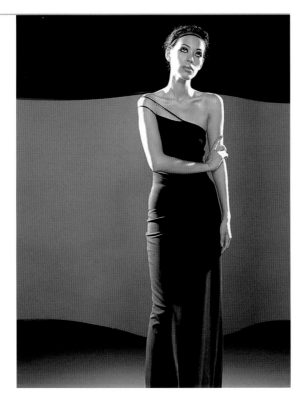

Assumption of the Virgin into heaven, or the quiet dyer in Taipei single-handedly keeping alive the world's most ancient silk-colouring technique, in Asia, these aren't about fashion design, they are about culture design.

Old Gods in New Bodies

Beyond its love of impressions and images, Asian fashion thinking is permeated by an influence that is irrelevant in the West: religion. All of the spiritual identities that dominate the imagery of Asian religions – Taoist, Buddhist, Hindu, Muslim, Christian – derive from societies stabilized by religious devotions, class mythologies and ancestral bonds.

Clothing is devotionalism for the body. The Chinese cheongsam, the Indian sari and *salwar kameez* and the Malay *baju* and sarong are like altar devotions. They decorate by casting complexity upon simplicity. They preserve rigidities of form. They stylize into abstraction the primal emblems of their spiritual reachings. The Malaysian and Indonesian woman's formal garb of today originated in the god-king's (*rajadeva*) of the region's distant Hindu past. Luxuriantly garbed Lakshmis and Kuan-Yins are nourished each day with sticks of smoking incense, thimble-sized tumblers of water and tea. Whether housed in the Hindu *kovil* or the Chinese dragon house under a tree, within you find a gold figure dressed in gold cloth.

For in Asia to cloak is to reveal – not the physical self, but rather the mind and spirit self as spoken through the rhythm of stride, bearing and gait. Out of the cheongsam, salwar, sheath, A-line and flounce, Asian fashion designers create grace, vigour, nobility, imitativeness and girlishness. Indonesia is the tribal wear of the rice culture greeting that of the after-five culture. Singapore is like living within a bolt of sheer silk. Malaysia shimmers the body into a mix of aviary and botanical garden. With the reserved Thai woman, there is always more to be discovered and, once you do, you can't get enough of her. The Catholic intensity of the Philippines conjures palettes so saturated that they outcolour a cardinal's crimson robes. Taiwanese women see purity in their ancestry and want it on their bodies. Hong Kong fashion is the art of the Tang dynasty made wholly contemporary. The modern women of China are happily discovering the multitude of ways they can express themselves in their clothing. There is a single quality in each of these women. They allow you to think you're seducing them. But by getting you to think that, they have already seduced you.

Indonesia
Noni Tawangsari – **Somewhere above the Sky**

Design by Sebastian Gunawan

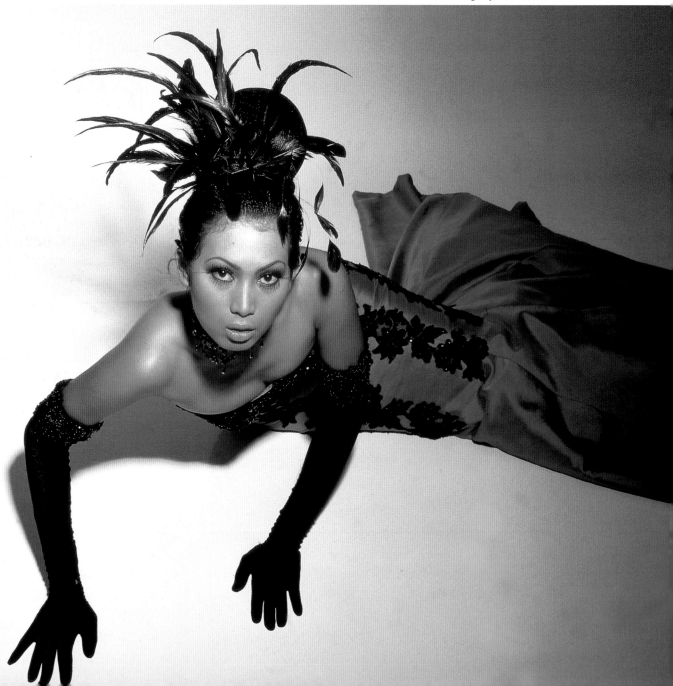

Jakarta's shopping malls blend the verisimilitude of cityscape solids with a fabric aviary. Primary colours of yellow and red and green and blue. Secondary hues of primaries merged together – browns, pinks, maroons, fuchsias and tangerines. Tertiary tints mixed of two secondaries – wedgwood, orchid, quail's egg, putty, taupe. Sky hues above and earthly tints below.

In Indonesia, the truths of a woman are hidden by the drape, form and movement of her garb. Beauty's veils reveal beauty itself. Her clothes embrace the symbols of religion, temple, hearth. But they are much more than that. The ideals we see so often motivating Indonesian garments are those of the theatre.

A woman's wear marries self and city in such a way that she becomes part of a modern urban tribe, which is little removed, except in modernities such as technology and banking, from the tribes that once peopled the island's forests and towns. Like the garments of old, the modern Indonesian woman ornaments herself, exposes her inner beliefs, expresses her loves – all more or less at once. If we look beneath the decorative sensations into the universal symbols of who she is presenting herself to be, we see that she is the past giving new life to the present. She is a mother, and that comes before her social standing and her wealth.

In Indonesia, clothing was once a defence against uncertainty. It summoned the aid of the protective forces that live *noni tawangsari,* somewhere above the sky. Bad harvests, poor weather, the fish not biting, unexpected outbursts of thunder and lightning, volcanoes, a still-born child. All could be protected against by veils. Masks.

The rules of life were strict. They had to be in order to preserve the limited supply of luck. Hence, in most of life's events, tensions were left unrevealed. Food was shared with good humour, even when there wasn't enough of it. Rites of passage were accomplished without enslaving their beneficiaries to debt. People laughed a lot. And they cried a lot.

And so, too, they veiled. What you see is what you don't see; it is what you are supposed to see. Almost everywhere in Indonesia the costume of the dance, especially the mask, is inseparable from the dance itself. Dance invokes the goodness of the gods. Masks communicate with higher powers, reinforce welfare and safety, and repel the evil forces that cause calamities.

Today the mall is the dance. The archipelago's abundant techniques intended to transform cloth into something else – and thus veil woman – are no different in the mall than time out of mind ago. The techniques of folding, binding, clamping, crimping, knotting, and sewing. *Ikat* and batik and *prada.* Embroidery, beading, *gringseng.* Tie-dye, clamp-resist, *tritik, plangi, bandha.* Stitch-resistant with overdyes, hand-painted and machine-printed, embroidered. Silver- and gold-leafed. Delicacies of nature. Abstract blots of city.

A bit of urbanity never hurt a good myth.

Didi Budiardjo

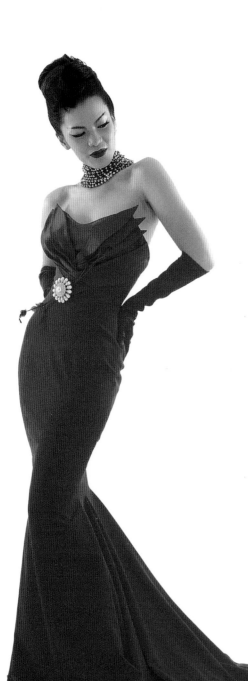

In unimaginable juxtapositions of colour – copper, umber, olive, turquoise and salmon, fawn, teal, flax – Didi's tints dominate an after-five or evening event. He is a study in collective consciousness, a mix of art and psyche. The result is a cheery navigation through yesteryear redolence that retains the exoticism of the Kingdom of Solo while discarding its starch.

Although he does fine things in his Anonymous line with powder-blue lace and silk at as little as a third of the couture price, it is his exoticism that stirs the imagination, his combining black lace on a white bustier attached to a skirt of Italian and Chinese embroidery. Sometimes his unusual relationships are pure felicity – the psychology of a splendid jewel on a simple dress is an ancient notion that, via Didi, is preserved virtually intact.

"My clients come to me with a basic problem: 'I have nothing to wear for this event.' Then they describe the things they like and don't like – what colours they can't or won't wear, the kind of accessories they like and so on. I show them fabrics, we talk about colours. Sometimes I do a sketch, but with most of my regular clients we just work with the fabrics, developing the garment's basic look as we go along. I think of what she's going to be doing when she wears the garment, her movements, the

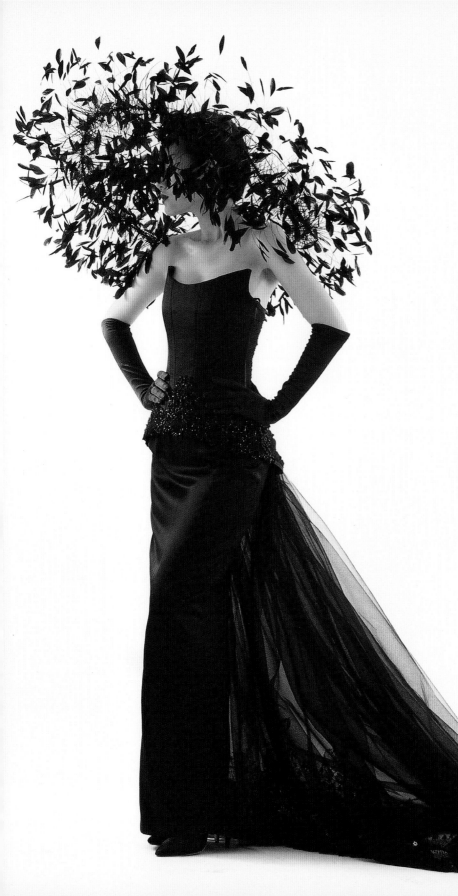

"From childhood
I learned about the
symbiotic relationship
between the architect
and the builder.
I found the same
symbiosis between
myself as fabric
designer and my
weavers, between
myself as fashion artist
and my customers as
fashion wearers."

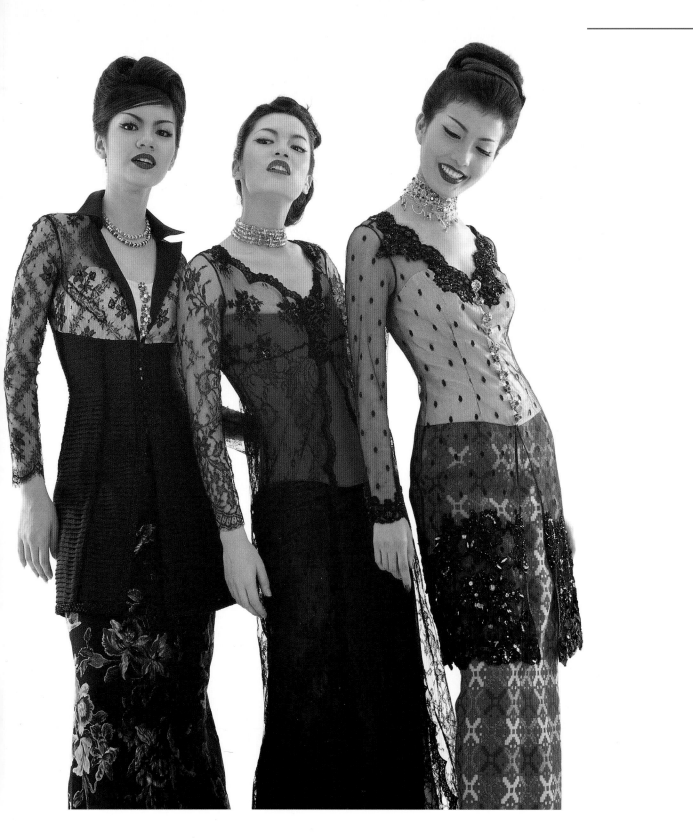

"To me, proportion is a lot more interesting than effect for effect's sake. I like to suggest rather than state."

angles from which she will be seen – say, at a reception, a buffet table, sitting for tea, dancing.

Beyond the close working relationship with the client, what inspires me to design the way I do? There is no one thing that consistently inspires me, a 'muse' so to say. Fantasy attracts me. Things that are not very real. Seeing a piece of really interesting fabric always gets me excited – especially colour, but also texture, drape, movement, the behaviour of a fabric. Surprisingly, the material itself does not often inspire an actual design. Other things do that, like the shape of a line I see on the street or in an ad or a movie, for example. Many times I am half way through thinking about a garment when I decide on the fabric to use.

While I like to keep things minimal, I also feel the need to make a design striking in some way. One option is to put an area of high detail on a dress that is basically unadorned – speckles of beading at the shoulders or bust, for example, or off-centred beadwork on one side for a vanishing cloud effect. Asymmetry can work wonders on a body that's not particularly shapely. In my beadwork I stay away from getting too brocade-like. "

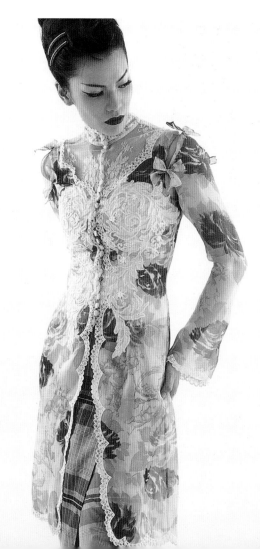

"Colour alone does not always make a great garment. I put colours and complex weaves on clean, simple forms, to create elegant designs that really turn heads."

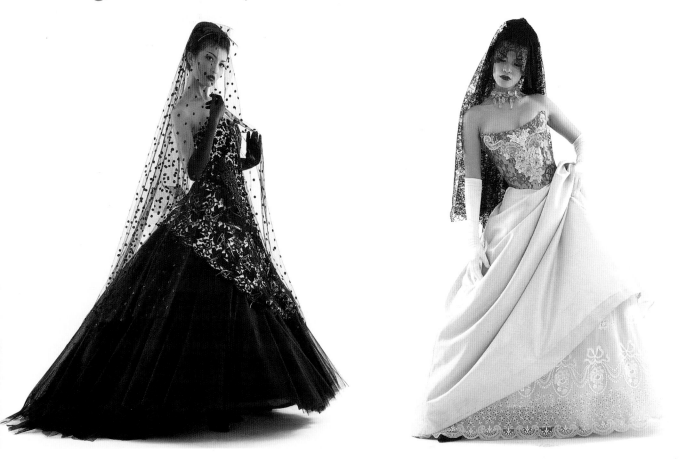

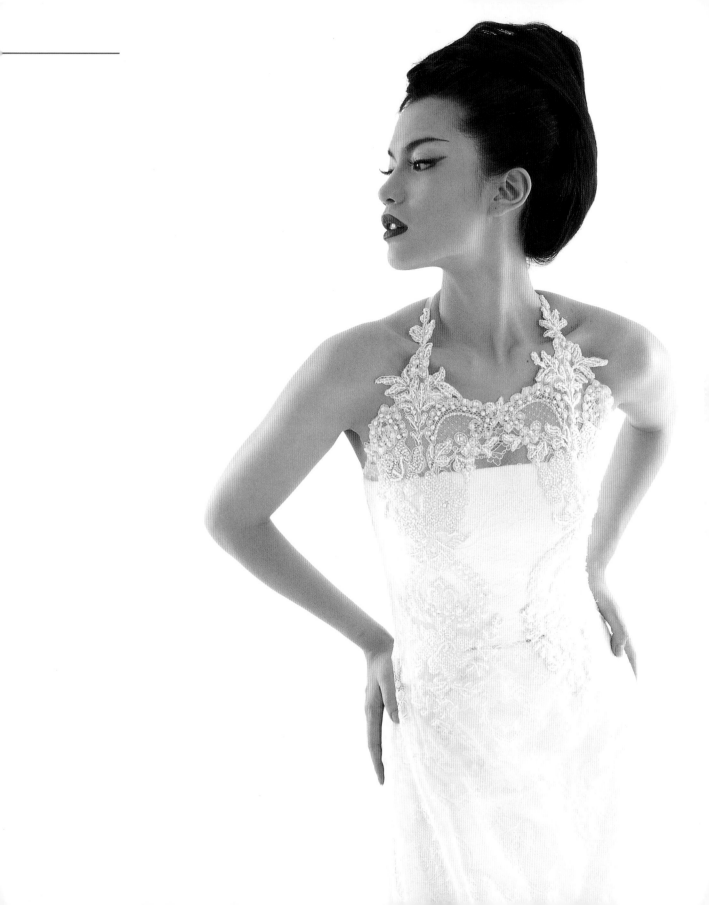

Carmanita
Indonesia

As a contemplation of the visual, Carmanita's work is surpassed only by the variety of Indonesia itself. In these isles, there is considerable precedent for masks that reveal by concealing. She, too, uses the mask. The garment's beginning is mood. Its memories are of another life, a visual perfume of colour, splendour, character, personality, fabric, integrity.

"The sources of my images are so multilayered that it is difficult to sort them out. They are internal and external, organic and geometric. They come from inspirations as varied as spiders' threads, snails' tracks, leaves, stones, sticks, rope, eggs, spirals, triangles, arrows, moons, circles, crescents, snakes, dissected rectangles, lines with wings, fire, lumps, moving water, star patterns, bones, music, drums, the songs of Indonesia's many forgotten tribes far away in the hidden valleys.

We are time capsules of memories that move us from place to place. We are the inner spirit behind all that is around us.

Java is deep, rich, hidden, sensuous. There are hierarchies of language, levels of meaning that you discover in the backyard gardens, getting water at the fountains. It can be like living in an old family photo album come to life: the wise old women, the batik makers, the traditional colours, the browns and oranges, and how they dye them. My art is trying to capture the mystical atmosphere of ancient Solo, its air of princesses, Hindu and Buddhist beliefs, Islam and animism, all mixing into the spirit of people, their memories, the pace at which they move.

The Indonesian woman's life is an elaborate, stunning, slow unmasking of her self, the divesting of the complex elaborations that encrust her from childhood throughout her life. It is only in her fifties that she can shed her old costume and emerge as a woman of revelation. At the end of her life, she is the self she was at birth, but strengthened and coloured to become the self she is now. Like the ancient tribes of Indonesia which originated all of these psychologies. Like the villages where the old and the new are the same. Like Indonesia. Like my designs. Like me."

"Earth my body. Water my blood.
Air my breath. Fire my spirit."

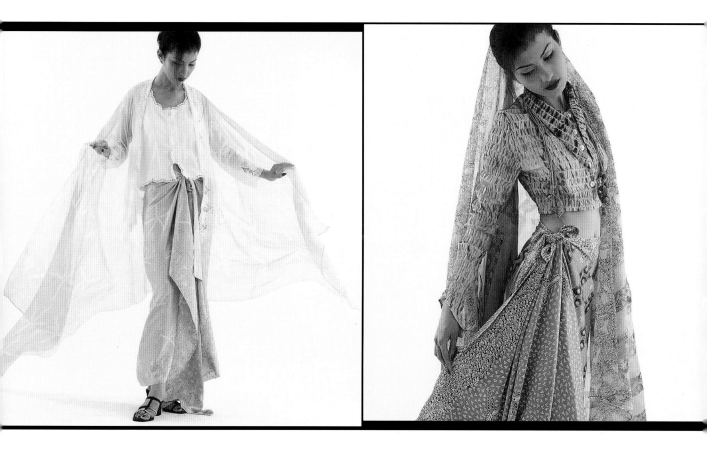

"I try to combine the tribalist with the
fine artist, the spiritual with the intellectual.
I am married to both of these worlds.
That's why my works are wall hangings
as well as garments."

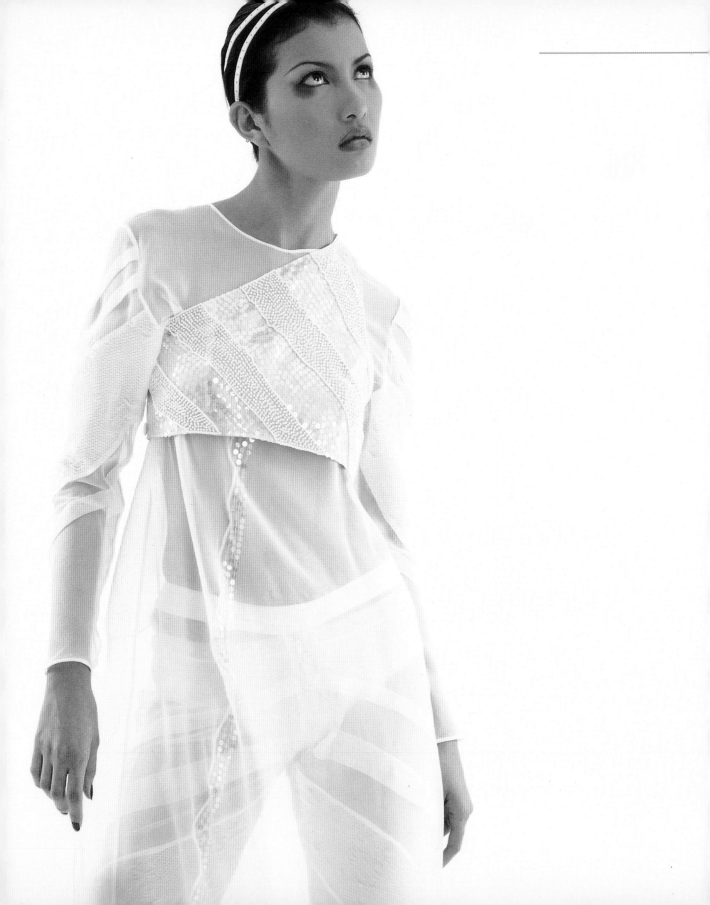

Ronald Gaghana
Indonesia

Out on to the table they come, a seemingly endless array of colour-laden weaves. Madder red, verdigris, umber, robin's egg, woad as blue as the windows of Chartres cathedral. Ronald Gaghana's Elements line plays colours like a piccolo plays notes: clear, penetrating, emotional. Soft brights like salmon and turquoise, sunflower and coral. Bronze for a summery feel. Black for drama. Rich textures in beiges and light browns. White illusions in chiffon and androgynous fabrics. Anthracite-coloured fabric interwoven with a subtle juxtaposition of hummingbird blue and the silvery blue of the overhead sky at sunrise. Zigzagging across these are pencil-wide strips of salmon and matchstick-wide lengths of saffron. He's young. He's also good.

"Reality is no aphrodisiac. I try to give the wearer as much latitude as possible. Fabric, like the body, is a fluid medium. Once I establish the curve and flow of one part of the body with the fluidity and drape of the cloth, the fabric then flatters the other parts. Then I can alter colours and detail, but the flattery remains.

But drape is very fabric-specific. What works well with linen can be a catastrophe with wool. Jersey and crêpe resemble each other, but they define the body very differently. Simplicity does not exclude voluptuousness.

Once I have the chosen the fabric, I work out the colours. Usually I start with one colour that I sense to be right for the garment and the occasion, then work outwards from there. I tend to put no more than two shades into a garment, contrasting a more vivid hue with a subtle colour. The eye is always eager for new images and nothing attracts the eye like interesting contrasts.

I spend a great deal of time in direct contact with each piece. It is essential that my garments feel wonderful on the body of the wearer. A woman reflects the patterns in her garments. If she wears scallop shells, she becomes a tropical sea. Flowers, and she's a garden. Clouds, and she's endless change.

Every technique imparts its own beauty. The challenge comes from assembling their energies, exploring their nuances, exhausting every possibility, learning how to control them without stifling their imaginativeness.

In Jakarta, we made-to-order designers do things our own way. We keep our businesses big enough to live off but small enough not to lose direction. Once a fashion business gets a certain size, it tends to gain identity but lose quality."

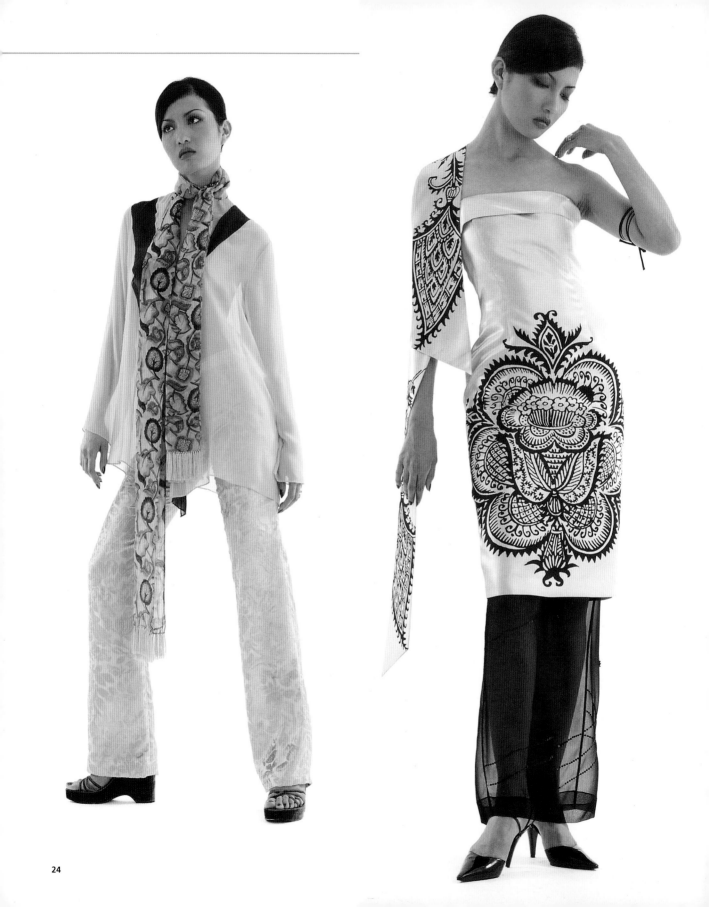

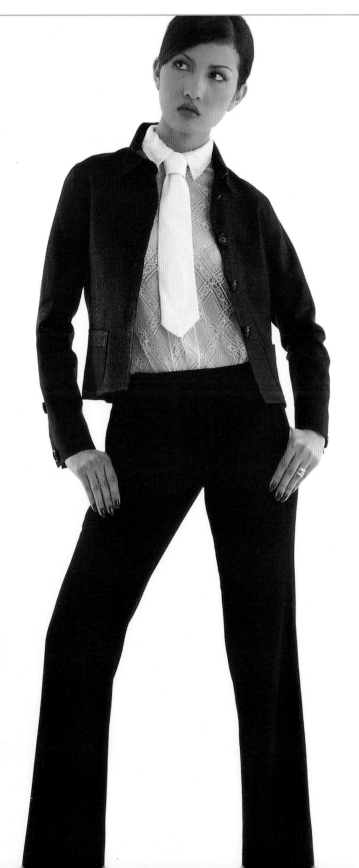

"My work concerns itself with the finesse that tailoring brings a garment."

Sebastian Gunawan
Indonesia

Sebastian Gunawan's Pret-a-Port line of transparent chiffons and lace can do marvels with the peekaboo look. However, his work isn't for the two-dimensional remoteness of the mannequin behind the window; it is for the three dimensions of a woman's body and the inexhaustibly larger dimension of the woman's self.

Since most visitors to a designer's atelier soon tire of long elaborations on the subject of manufacturing techniques, Sebastian gracefully adds descriptions of the human dimension: the dilemmas of designing for production; the exacting demands of catalogue printing; and how he knows when to change the many hats he must wear.

"I became interested in fashion design when I saw some dresses in an international fashion magazine. I was struck by the idea that clothes can be beautiful with or without the woman. My parents were artistically sensitive, so I already knew about seeing ordinary things as beautiful.

From very early on I was inspired by drama and glamour. I've always been a dramatic designer. But even when I create dramatic garments, I still include touches of the commercial.

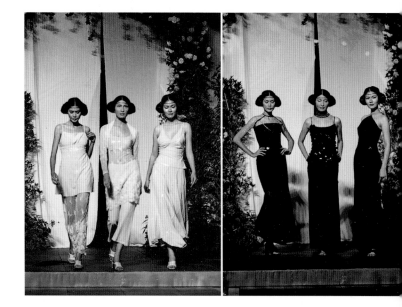

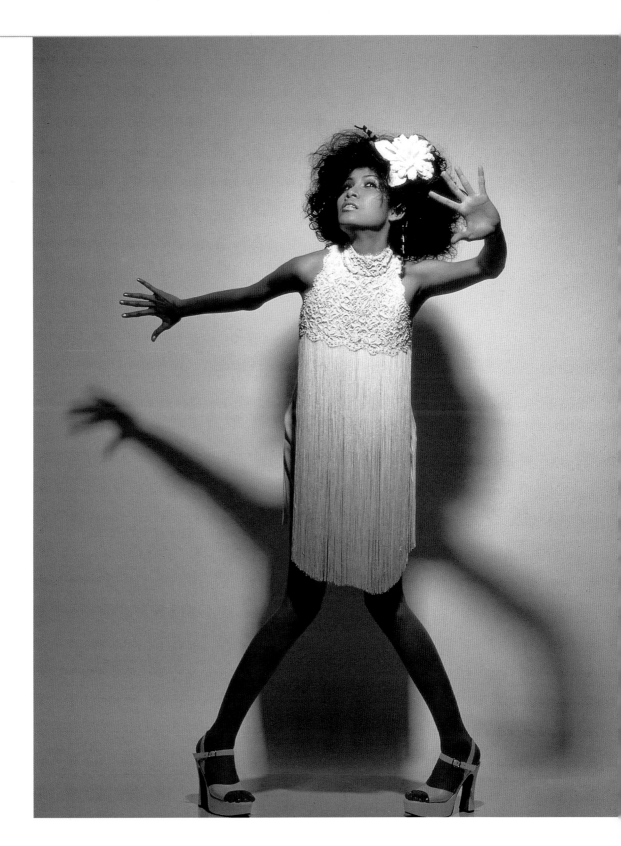

"I design in such a way that when you look at one of my dresses, you can't imagine how it was made. I get a thrill out of looking like I've achieved the impossible."

After years of travelling and seeing how couturiers operate, my work today is still based on what I feel inside. Hiding beautiful things inside plain surfaces has always been a fascination. Even when I make a basic black suit, I do something like put in an extraordinary lining you don't see from the outside, like the bird whose brilliant colour isn't revealed until it spreads its wings.

There's something internal about fashion design, something deep inside me that can't be explained. It is that which motivates me. I feel I'm part of a gigantic, exotic, gorgeous machine. Daily life doesn't give most people the courage to be the things they really want to be, so I give them courage through their clothes.

Like everyone, I have my signature motifs – oriental, exotic, highly layered. Every dress has to have its own theme. I'm inspired most by shape and concept. Only then do I look for a fabric to achieve them. I like the detailed look, the made-by-hand look, the mosaic look, the embroidered look. The greatest delight I take in my designs comes from their drama, the different ways of expressing, accessorizing, texturing. **"**

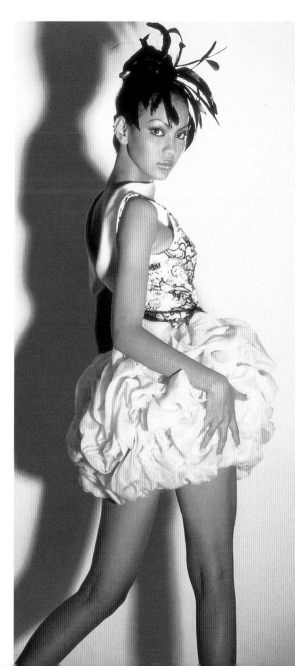

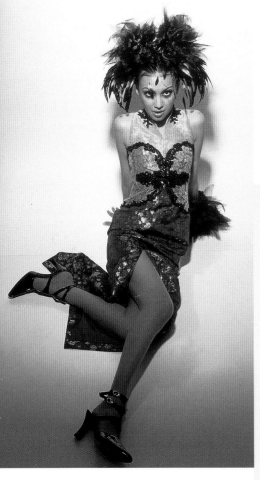

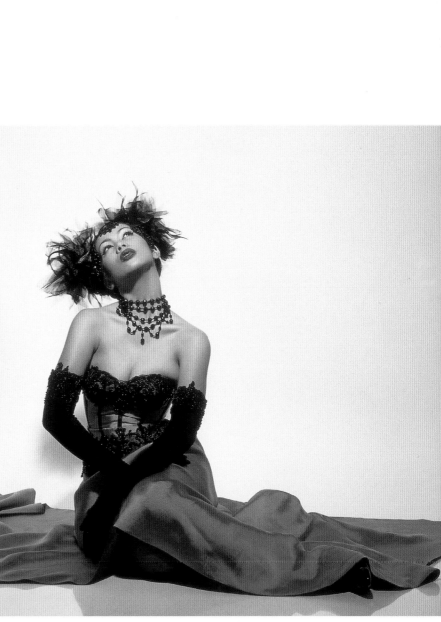

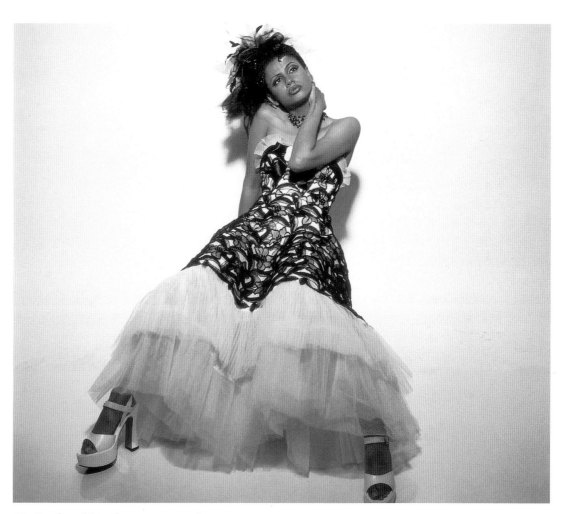

"Of all things that go into a garment, colour is the most important. I want colour to exist not only on the surface, but saturated all through the material, to the point that it penetrates and colours the wearer."

Ghea Panggabean
Indonesia

Ghea unites the world's artefacts into a single artistic vision – a Gaia of the art force, so to pun. Setting forth on the female river of fecundity, Ghea's goal is to create a style that unites history and art with the latest codes in business and contemporary wear. 'I try to create a way for a woman to communicate her awareness that something in her, and in her view of the world, is timeless.'

"I am known as someone who has discovered many new ways of using handmade textiles and ancient motifs from the Indonesian textile tradition. I am a funnel from the past to the present. I believe something eternal exists in things of great beauty and that people transcend their character because of it. Fashion exists wherever enough people grasp its essentials: elegance, style, quality, craftsmanship, detail, attention to the wearer, exquisiteness, innovation, materials. It is a kind of courageousness to not care about the marketplace, to explore the boundaries of fabric and fabrication, and then go beyond them.

My medium is thread, but I work with womankind. I want to create designs that combine the past and the future in a continuum of the present, in the same way that clothing is as contemporary as the present day and yet the most ancient of art forms. Some people sense that urge towards enormous human continuity when they walk into a cathedral, others when they experience the age-old cultures one finds in Asia or Iran or Morocco. For me, when the wearer puts on the garment and it expresses everything I wanted it to, yet has taken on something more, that is magic. Then I'm at one with every clothing maker who ever was.

The woman I design for is sensitive to fabric, to material handled in an unusual way. She is unafraid of the spotlight. She enjoys a substantial amount of detailing and personal embellishment in her clothes. I design what she needs to nourish all of her being: her intellect, her femininity, her sensuality, her sense of daring.

Designing is like dancing. My partner, the fabric, has its own energy, its own expression. It creates something separate from my creativity. If I'm willing to take chances, the results can surprise me and be truly extraordinary.

If we created no future in our work, who would? My garments are the life force waiting to be worn. The antiquity and continuity of cloth is so vital in today's rush of the impermanent."

"We Indonesians are heirs to a tradition of colour whose heritage is so distant that it was already far advanced by the time it was first painted on pots and dyed into threads."

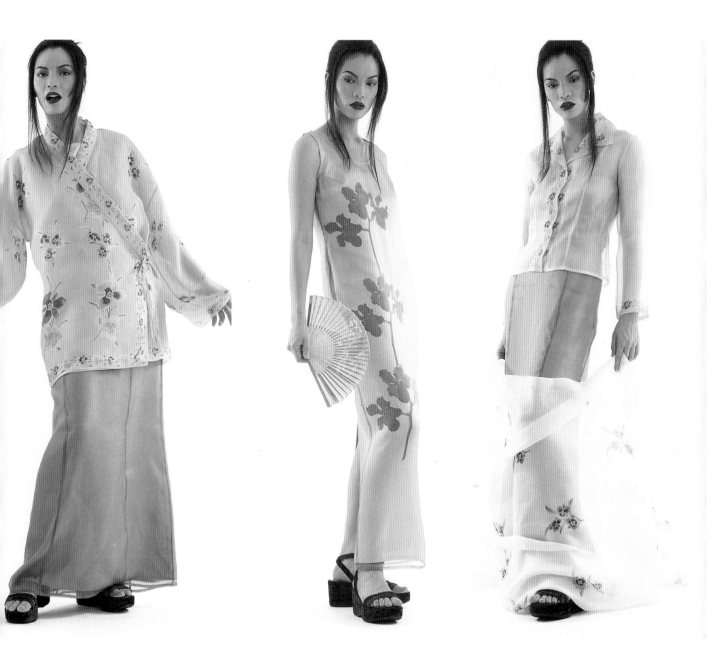

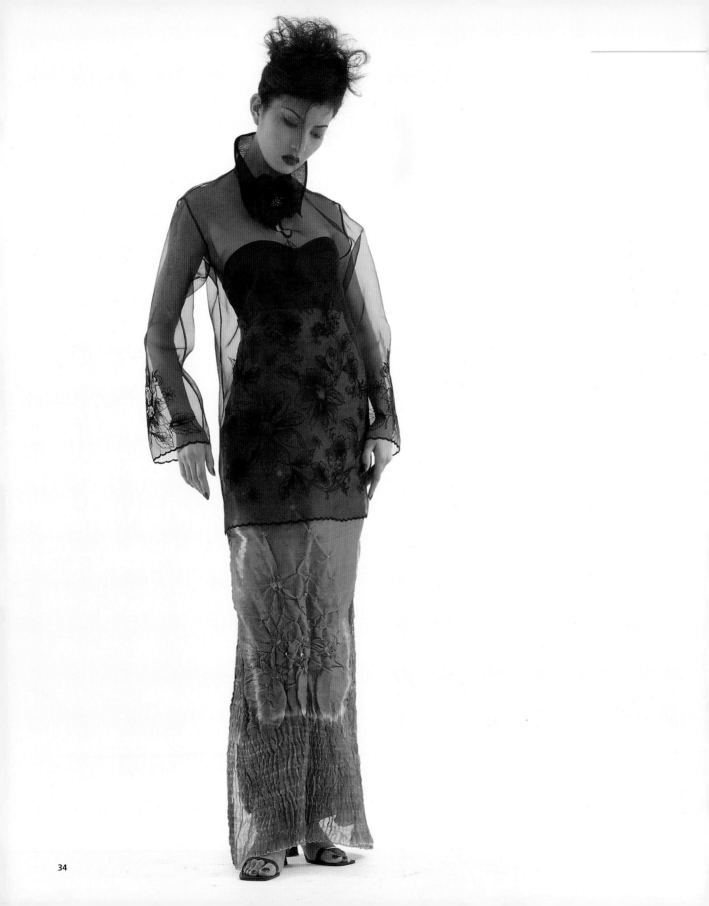

House of Prajudi
Indonesia

Indonesian fashion does little borrowing and the international names that crop up are few and far between. Even within the country, designers have little influence on each other, since there is so much local colour to draw upon.

Prajudi Admodirdjo's elegant ready-to-wear set the standard for quality fabrication in Indonesia for a long time – a discipline which many others have emulated. Some say his work reflected the difference between the designers of his generation, who largely studied in Germany, and the younger ones of today, who study mainly in Italy and London. Yet, in both cases, the vividness of local sensibility demonstrates how vaporous internationalism can be when facing such rich internal cohesiveness.

Sadly, Prajudi himself passed away abruptly in 1996, but his legacy is being carried on today by the capable hands of Mr Ari Saputra. The fact that internal integrity can transfer so quickly and successfully from one designer to another says much about the spirit of art in Indonesia, the sense that the self is but a thread. It is, after all, the House of Prajudi.

Prajudi Admodirdjo died at the peak of a career that doubtless would have gone on for decades longer. Instead of an interview, we have therefore substituted information from his atelier about his life and thinking.

Prajudi Admodirdjo left Jakarta in 1970 to study architecture in Germany. After eight months he changed to study dress design and fashion.

In late 1972, he returned to Indonesia to work on his own. That same year Queen Juliana of the Netherlands made a state visit to Indonesia and Prajudi was given the honour of presenting a design for her. Impressed palace circles then opened doors for him to design the attire for state guests.

In 1975 he established Studio One with two of his friends. This venture focused on ready-to-wear garments using the then somewhat unfashionable technique of batik design, turning it into the innovative vehicle of quality and style that marks Indonesian batiks today.

In 1978 Prajudi decided to concentrate more on his couture business. He built one of the most sophisticated and exclusive fashion houses in Indonesia. His elegant creations brought considerable international influence into Indonesian design thinking.

"Our clothes should have both immediacy and timelessness. The House of Prajudi tries to achieve this with layered looks, fluid transparencies, uniting the simple and the complex with childlike images and delicate intimacy."

Prajudi's style is associated with the sophisticated pattern precision which typified the country's many local design traditions. His enthusiasm for Indonesia's culture led him to take part in backing a government programme to promote small-scale textile industries. His efforts came to focus on revitalizing the island's extremely rich tradition of ikat cloth manufacture. He devoted the same energetic support to abstract pattern weaving traditions in Siabu, to the glittering *tapis* cloth of Lampung, as well as to more established batiks.

Prajudi also contributed to the traditional costume of the country. The widely copied *kebaya Prajudi,* a modernized double-sheath woman's *kebaya* with puffed diagonally pleated sleeves, is one example of how his contemporary styling ideas reinterpreted traditional designs.

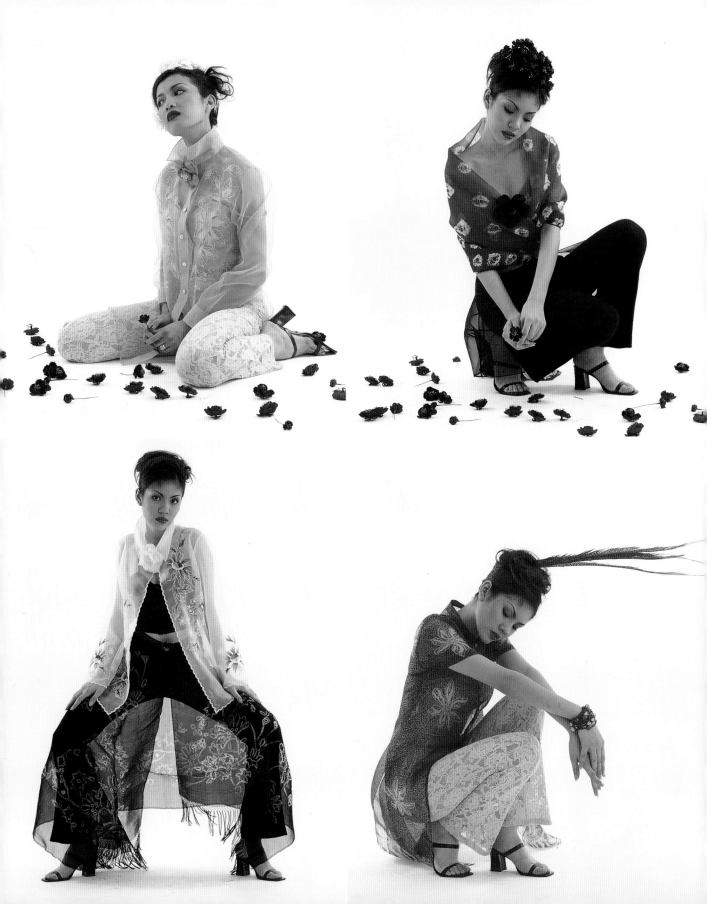

Lily Salim

**Lily Salim is Indonesia's Martha Graham.
She both looks and acts the part.
Drape plays a large role in her work,
for drape is the emotion of a fabric,
just as intensity was Martha Graham's
emotion of the dance. Yet Lily's chaste,
reserved look is like no other dance;
it is truly unique.**

"Much of my work is based on what I like
to wear. I am fascinated with the limitless
magic that happens when the flat surface
of a fabric transmutes to a moving three-
dimensional woman.

The body is an argumentative medium.
Once you've got the curve and flow of one
part of the body to agree with the fluidity of

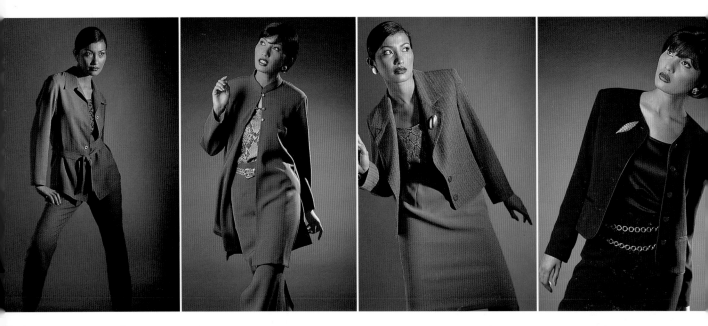

the cloth, the other parts of the body might then refuse. Body shape can be both the djinn and the genie in the designer's life – and often both at once. Hence jackets are designed to work from the shoulder line, blouses from the bust line, trousers from the hip.

The way a woman moves, which depends on what she's doing, determines where a garment should touch her body. Hence for me, activity directs design. I always begin with a specific garment in mind, with its own configuration of shoulders, hems, sleeves. I conceive of the body in the sculptural sense, with the woman's body as the armature. With a vague concept of the garment I want, I put a piece of cloth in front of me and then work without hesitation.

I love transmuting emotions into cloth. I have to love the feel of the materials I work with. I spend a great deal of time in direct contact with each piece. Sometimes it is hard to tell who's really in charge, me or the fabric. The fabric flows, the drape flows, the body flows. Then the garment is finished, bought and worn. It flows around a body. Its intricacies and ornaments are at once revealed and hidden. It turns an occasion into a ceremony. It blends the wearer's personality with my personality while retaining the uniqueness of each.

It's not easy. Many years of experience help. **"**

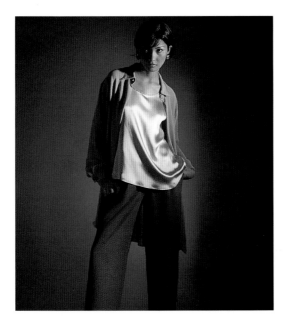

"My ideal is to keep clothes very simple, easy to wear. Practical, so you can wear them in any place, at any time."

Biyan Wanaatmadja

Indonesia

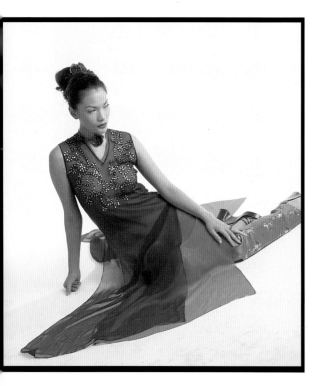

Fashion is the portrait of a class within a snapshot of the times. In our era of mass-manufactured clothing, with five fashion seasons a year and polyester-princess advertisements, the costume tradition has been overlooked to the extent that it's almost been lost. We're supposed not only to look like the model in the ad, but to want to look like her.

Biyan dresses a large number of women who design for themselves. It is almost a canon among his clientele that a good body without a good design is like a good design without a good body. His customers are therefore much more demanding about cut and finish than buyers in other parts of the world. Biyan has become a master of subtleties, such as the effect that asymmetry can have on a line or that an off-centre cut can have on a hip. He knows that there's nothing better than black near the waist of an Asian black-haired beauty, or that a bit of rhinestone never hurt a deliciously cool silk.

He knows how to structure loosely below the waist and tighter above. He likes comfort and clean lines, the easy drape of fabric cut on the bias. His is the subtle kind of chic you can wear at home, on a Sunday stroll along the beach, or on a flight to Mauritius for a holiday.

"A woman can't be defined. She knows that if there's a competition for attention between herself and the garment, it is she who must win. She must not be shy."

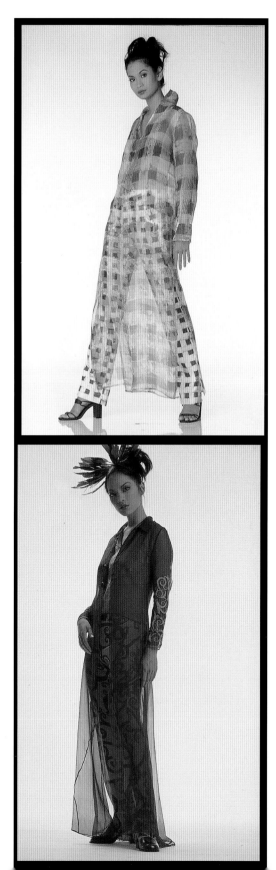

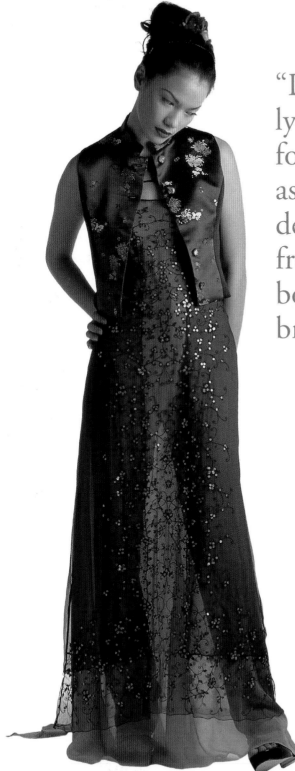

"Design is essentially lyrical. It doesn't exist for itself. It exists as the child exists, delighting in the freedom of being bold, being vivid, bright and free."

"I started making my own clothes when I was very young, playing with the cloth in Mom's fabric bin. Finally she cut a pattern and told me to go ahead. The first thing I made was a shirt. I learned to sew by tacking hems, then finishing dresses with my Mom. I didn't have colouring books, so I mentally coloured clothes instead.

The first time the notion of pure form came to me was when I discovered Balenciaga, how he draped, how he sculptured. I began to notice how the sloping shoulders of the Twenties contrasted with the chunky shoulders of the Forties, how business suits for women would minimize the waist and flatten the bosom during good economic times and do the opposite during bad. I noticed how one can emphasize or de-emphasize the silhouette by a different cut of fabric.

Fabric's softness and elasticity evoke freedom. Fabric is the vehicle for everything: light, colour, motion, shape, texture, mood, emotion, intensity. The result is an inspiring variety of weave and colour and cut. We who design clothes never lack for something new to work on.

The only constant in fashion is change. In Asia the tastes for colours change often, so there are many opportunities to explore. So I experiment with draping, embroidery, beading, dyeing. I aim for a collection that is classic. I want something a person can wear five years from now and for it still to look original."

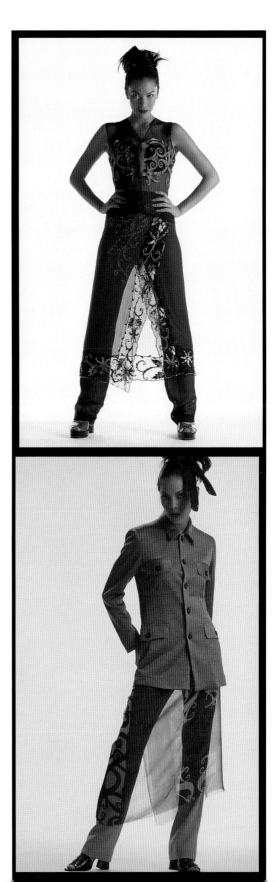

Singapore
Conspicuous Subtlety

Design by Esther Tay

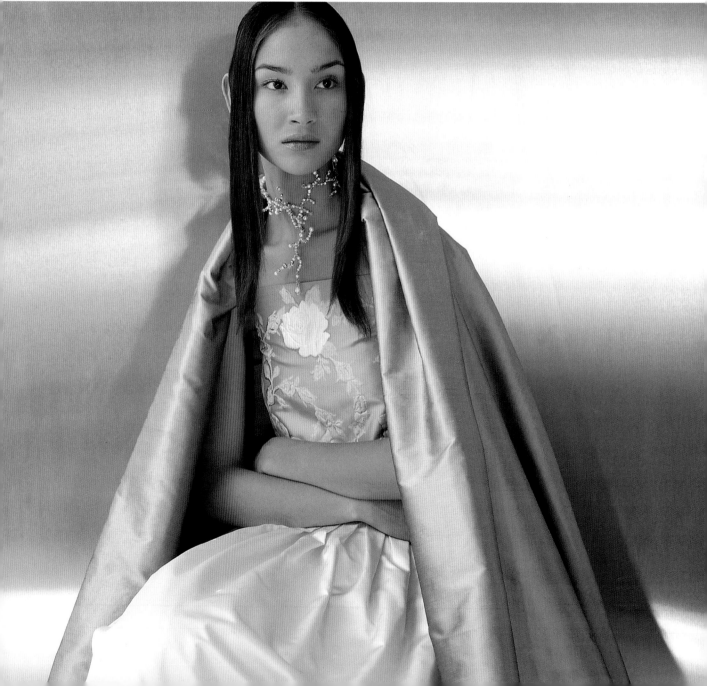

A conversation with a Singaporean fashion or interior designer consists of a little theory, a little self-revelation and a lot of shop talk. An hour with Esther Tay and her husband Paul Chua, with Wykidd Song, with Peter Teo, or with the Singapore fashion world's doyen behind the scenes Alan Koh provides a ready reply to the perennial question, 'Can reality ever be as interesting as fantasy?'

Singapore, on the surface at least, is about sun: people doing laps in the city's many swimming pools, bougainvillea flowers bursting from pots, jasmines cascading luxuriantly and fragrantly over walls and chirping colonies of birds. The air is one of self-confidence, luxury and middle-class contentment.

Pu Yen-t'u, one of the greatest early Chinese calligraphers made the following observations: 'The art of the visible invisible is what is needed. / The work must be mobile and vigorous – above all, banality must be banished. / The work must avoid falling into the obvious.' And where do you see these ideas today? Walking along Orchard Road.

Singapore is like a minimalist dance whose details are made all the more powerful by their subtlety.

As everywhere, the immediacies in life are the Singaporean's constant preoccupation – food, clothing, interiors, buildings, possessions, orderliness. Singapore is about forms of economy translated into forms of society.

For people accustomed to looking for art in everyday things, Singapore is the art that exists unseen within an infrastructure: the making of a city-state. No other city has the potential to become the Paris of Asia in the way that Singapore does.

Why Singapore? The Western press drubs this tidy isle over its forbidding the delights of chewing gum and spitting in the street. Others opine that business is the only culture in Singapore, that a successful business deal is the only self-expression people enjoy.

Nonsense. *Knowing* is the culture in Singapore. Singapore's most useful contribution to the world of the creative impulse is the idea that one originates by knowing what others don't.

As people undergo economic and cultural complexification, their sense for imagery simplifies. The details lessen until they arrive at a kind of psychically irreducible simplicity. This is the truth within the thing, the truth within the self. That's where Singapore is now.

Singapore's fashion designers understand the economic quality of vision, the wholeness that remains mostly unseen, in everything in the world that surrounds us. Now its artisans must deal with how to translate this into the shapes, forms, textures, smells, colours and juxtapositions of which fashion is made.

They understand that all things are wholes within a unity, that we can play with each of them, manipulate each of them, just as an artist masters the landscape of expression – grammar and vocabulary and the assembling of an image – to turn a city into history and a woman into light.

Allan Chai
Singapore

Allan Chai's fabric innovations combined with the marketing and management inventiveness of his long-time colleague Ross Chng comprise one of the several remarkable talent pairings that make Singapore unique in the fashion world. Like the city-state's other dynamic duos – Esther Tay and Paul Chua, Wykidd Song and Ann Kelly – a personal following coalesces around a unique fashion identity, which is translated into a retail following by building on a boutique-and-accessories identity.

"I once watched a watercolourist feathering in shadows cast by a gull in a seascape. It took him hours to do a few square inches. So too do my designs depend on hours of embellishment and detail if they are to be perfect.

I try to express two things in every work I do: the uniqueness of the wearer who buys it – nothing standard, nothing conventional, nothing held back – and of myself in creating it.

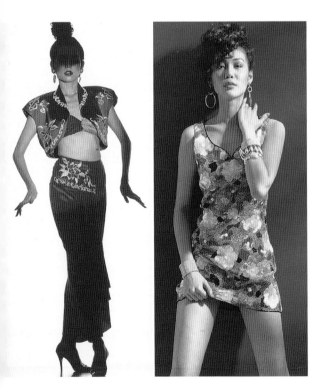

"In Singapore, I have been able to join the European and the oriental into something I can believe in."

To me, continuity is important, just as it is in the designs of Chanel or Issey Miyake. In them, you know what to anticipate. My continuity is in the fabric. That's what I drape.

I've never understood what kind of artist I am. I don't even ask. I just play with things and colours and shapes, and put them into patterns. I am not looking for results, I am playing with them. I can't leave simplicity alone. I keep adding things until a piece becomes my own. Design takes a lot of solitude. When I do it, I'm not very social.

I don't think of myself as exceptional. All this is given to me. I try not to get too attached to it. I know this season will pass. I design for the love of my work, not to impress or show. My images are for my own pleasure, but I also feel I am creating for a purpose greater than myself, to benefit others. That's my greatest good.

Working on a collection is a humbling experience. Design crosses borders, crosses time, crosses truths, crosses souls, to make sense of our surroundings. Design takes us away from ourselves by immersing us in the selves of others. "

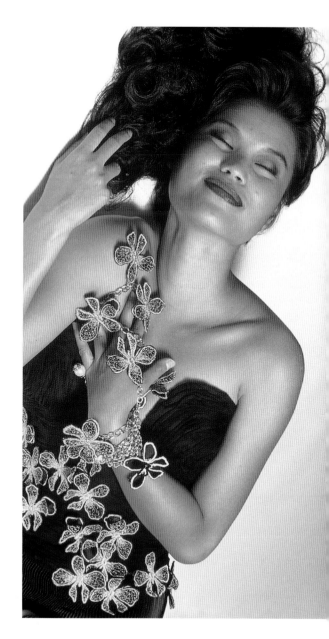

Celia Loe

Celia Loe is a prime example of the meritocratic mindset that drives Singapore so quickly forwards. Her creative contributions to the country's fashion industry have earned her no end of awards, including the Best Women's Wear Award at the Best of the Best Singapore Designer's Show. At the Association of South-East Asian Nations (ASEAN) Designers' Show in the Philippines, her clothes were featured in Elsa Klensch's *Style* programme aired on CNN.

Sometimes pure fashion doesn't always pay the bills, so she has also designed the uniforms for the Singapore Airlines subsidiary SilkAir; for the Post Office Savings Bank; for the Toa Payoh, Kandang Kerbau and Tan Tock Seng hospitals; for Tradewinds Tours; and for the Takashimaya department store.

"I've always designed clothes with a clean and uncluttered look. I try to help my buyers project their successful self-confidence and relaxed personality. The fashion designer's career is tough, yet its rewards are commensurably high.

Although I originally trained in London, in 1972 I came home to Singapore to set up my first factory and boutique. Today I travel frequently on sponsored fashion missions to Sydney, Paris, Tokyo, New York and London – places I did not dream of working in when I was just starting!

I have eight boutiques of my own, plus ten concessions in Singapore's leading department stores: Sogo, C.K. Tang and Takashimaya. Twelve years ago, I was the first Singapore designer to set up a boutique in the United Kingdom. In 1993, I opened a factory in Shanghai and I plan to open several retail outlets in the major cities of China.

Singapore has been good to me and I try to be good back. I sit on advisory committees in the Institute of Technical Education here and also in the Temasek Polytechnic's (Singapore) fashion and merchandising department. I also take on apprentices from such institutions for on-the-job training. I hope my vision of fashion's importance in Singapore's cultural life will be improved upon by the students and designers who are now rising up through the ranks on their way to launching their own careers."

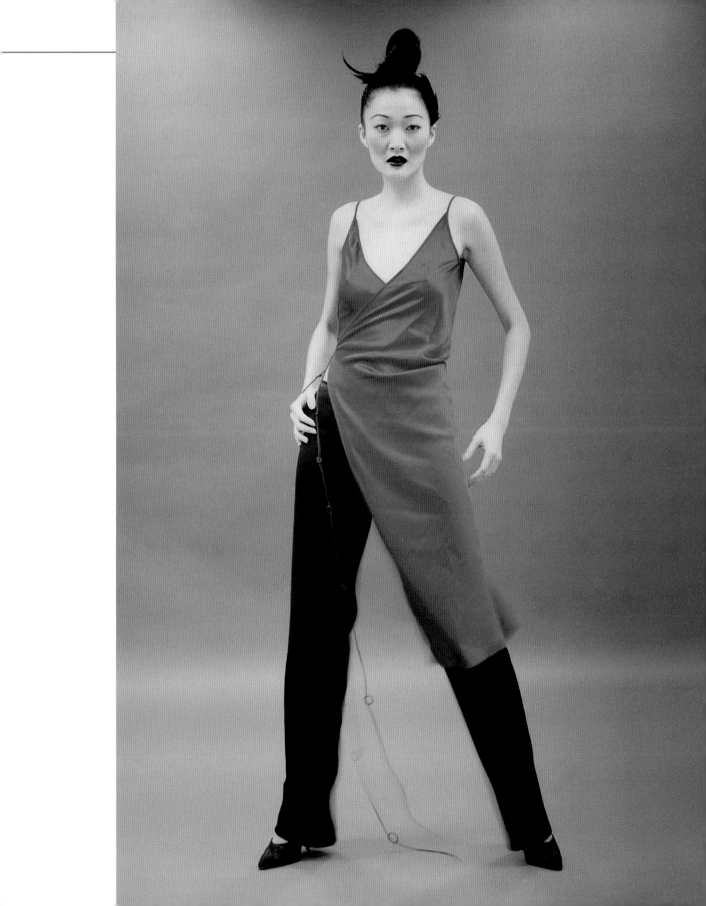

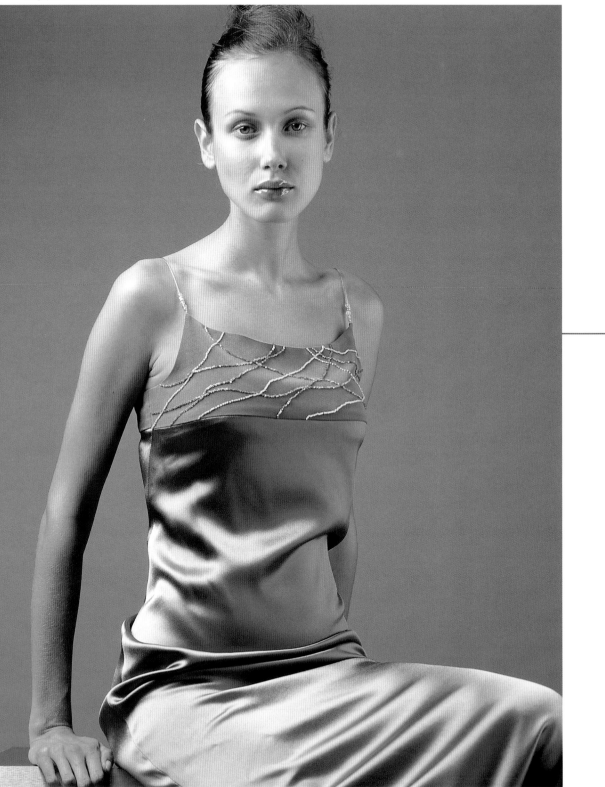

"For this book, I chose clothes that are soft, modern, elegant, and complemented by touches of unusual detailing."

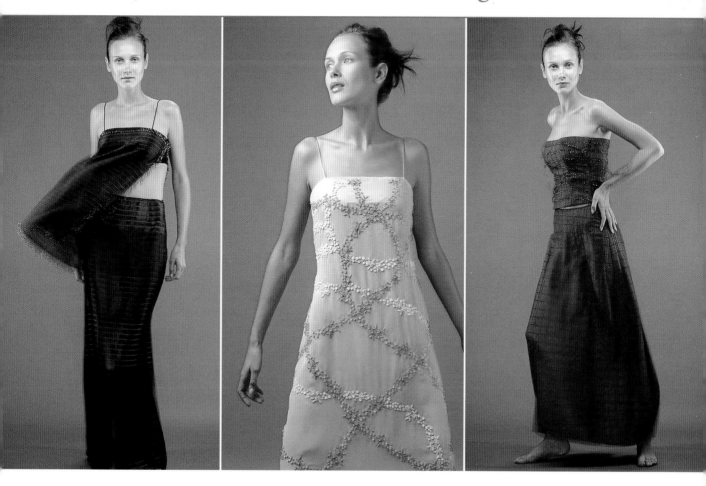

"The design
of a garment
should make
the woman
feel confident
and beautiful."

Cynthia Ng Meng Sim

Cynthia Ng is among the very young – indeed unproven – designers who abound in Asia. Compared with the paucity of training venues available to the more well-established designers in this book, Asia today is blossoming with design schools. Some are private, others part of formal degree courses on university curricula. Their shows – often sponsored by government textile promotion boards and presented as part of an annual textiles fair – reveal how differently today's young people create compared with the generation that is only ten years ahead of them. The tailoring tradition has far less influence and is being replaced by a fabric technology tradition.

Cynthia is a free-ranging structuralist who merges unusual shapes with unlikely materials. At so young a stage in her career, who knows what we'll be seeing from her in a decade. It certainly won't look anything like the work of the elder Singapore designers here. The minimalist look of today can't get any more minimal, so taste has nowhere else to go but towards the profusion of ideas simmering away in all those young heads.

"I started to get really interested in fashion when I was about thirteen. I wanted to be involved in the industry in some way, either as a designer, photographer, or journalist. I couldn't deny my love for fashion. I wanted to try to realize my dreams. At least I'll feel no regrets later in life.

I must have got my creative genes from my mother. She used to make her own clothes and most of the dresses for my sister and myself. When I was young, I loved to wrap myself in pieces of left-over fabric and fashion garments out of them. Using the same piece of cloth, I would create different designs and styles.

My design ideas are usually inspired by beautiful works of arts. This is probably due to my interest in music, photography, theatre, architecture, dance, paintings and literature.

I'm also inspired whenever I travel, which I love doing. I'm very curious to find out about the people and cultures of different countries, especially those whose lifestyles I could never imagine before I visited them.

I feel that fashion design is a form of art. I need to put a lot of thought into each design. It allows me to express myself. By understanding the design, one knows the designer."

Wykidd Song and Ann Kelly

Singapore

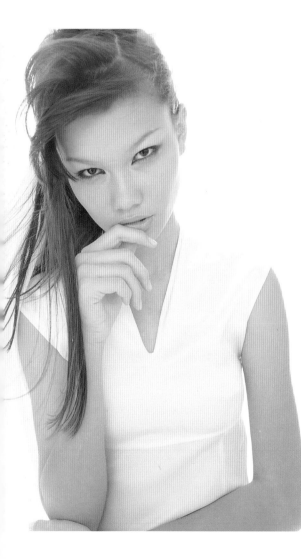

Wykidd Song and Ann Kelly are Singapore's fashion equivalent of I. M. Pei. They are the utter absence of artifice. Together they convey a sense of the wearer's complexity by reducing everything to its *serenissima,* its most serene self.

Song and Kelly unveil the classicism hiding behind every modernity. Their collections are timeless yet of the moment. Their understatement has a personality all of its own. They revere fine fabrics and have an unhesitating idea of how they should be used.

Their details are structural: texture, fabrication, tailoring, finish. Their sensibility is organic: feminine, modern, fluid. Their philosophy is purity and simplicity. Each collection reduces all that is extraneous to that which is both necessary and beautiful.

To them, Singapore is not a place for dressing down. Functional form is formal function. It all fits together.

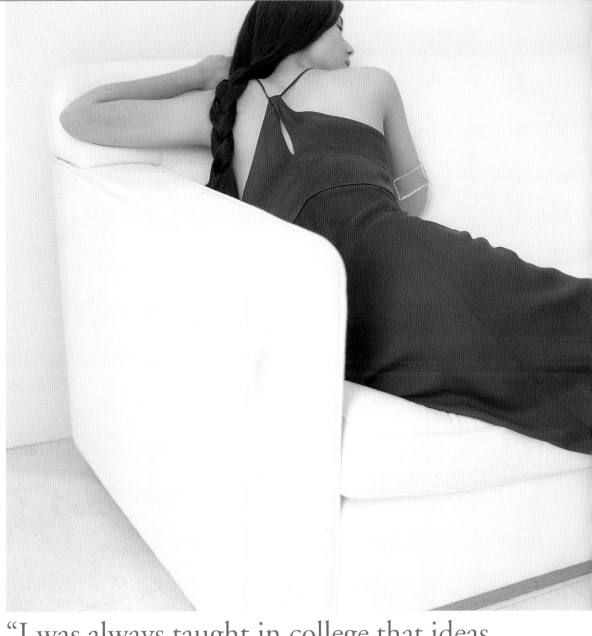

"I was always taught in college that ideas have to be developed. Then came real life and I found that they are intangible, not solid, even though a core is there."

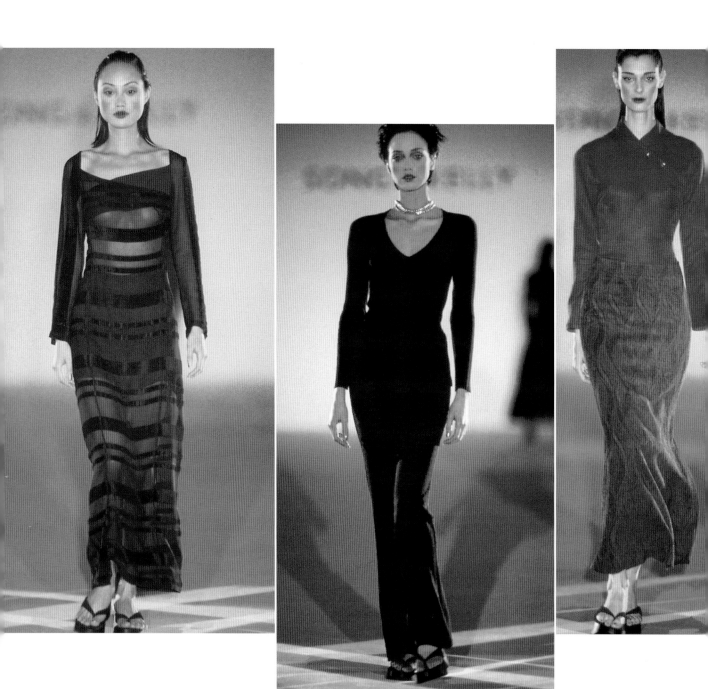

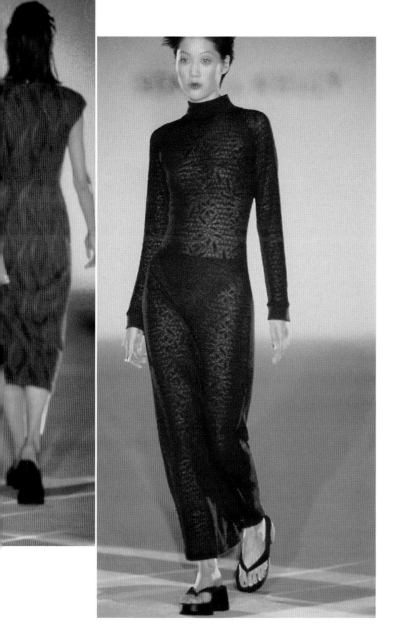

"We are a cross-cultural team that finds strength in our diversity. [Wykidd is a Singaporean who studied fashion in Britain. British-born Ann trained in graphic design.] We honed our experience in London, Milan and Hong Kong, and established Song & Kelly in 1994.

We see fashion as a business, but fashion creation as an art. Art has to sell to survive. Our design is an art of the Singaporean culture. We think this is what Singaporeans feel about their world. We don't mimic and we don't derive. Our style echoes the fusion of our backgrounds.

Our first idea is almost always the one that has staying power. Turning it into clothes takes a lot of collaboration. We bounce a lot of ideas off each other. We then catch them in the air and transport them on to paper. The star pieces are the one where we've conveyed our views to each other. It's a great reassurance when a couple in a store react to the pieces in the same way that we intended.

Our signature look is clean lines with a lot of structural details: feminine but strong, lots of opposites, strength in diversity. Opposites balance. Minimalism shows purity of detail. We are practical designers and our work must be wearable. The clothes must be simple but they must stand out. We isolate features, but we are so minimalist

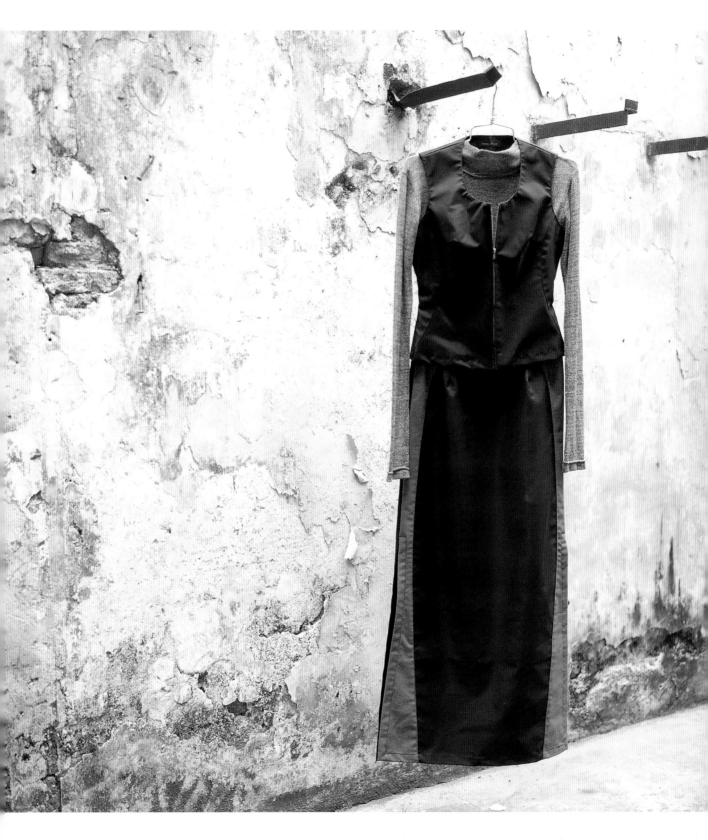

"Wykidd is very much inspired by photography – things like the way *National Geographic* handles forms in their photographs, the way they put different textures together. We do something of the same when we combine different fabrics."

that people tend to miss them, so we make sure they are obvious even though minimal. For example, we'll reverse a fabric where it seams, so the fabric faces outwards. The art is in seeing fabric as a graphic element, translating practical details into interesting forms, then taking away anything that is not useful.

There are inbuilt problems about Singaporean design that limit us internationally. Singapore has one season. People here don't take to cotton, wool and the other 'climate' fibres. Yet we have to design within the framework of the international seasonal convention – collections for spring, summer, fall and winter. This is partly because we sell internationally."

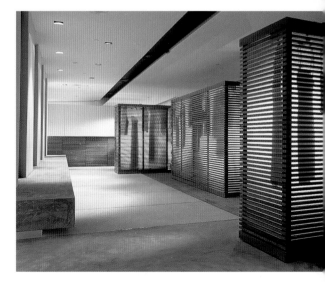

Esther Tay
Singapore

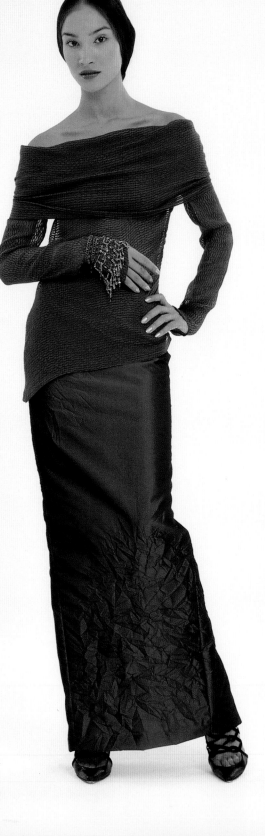

Inspiration – deep, soul-lifting inspiration – comes to Esther Tay while living or travelling in distant countries. Often her stimulus lies in the colour combinations she finds in country markets, in the sounds of people and animals, in celebrations and in the never-ending glances of the world's multitude of eyes. Along with heartbeats and lungs, she believes skin to be one of biology's greatest gifts of colour, just as the urge to wear colour is one of the greatest gifts of the soul.

"When I was young, I lived in a little village next to the sea. The sea inspired my sense for colour's endless variations. Silver and blue can do myriads of things together and yet still be silver and blue. Even now colour attracts my eye first. Then shape. Then texture. Then feel. Then form.

As long back as I can remember, I wanted things to be something else. Another colour, another shape. I began translating these desires into clothes when I apprenticed in a haberdashery shop for eighteen months. I was surrounded by textiles, so I looked for ways to use them. When I showed my first little 'collection' to my boss, she turned the haberdashery into a boutique and called it The Nutmeg Tree.

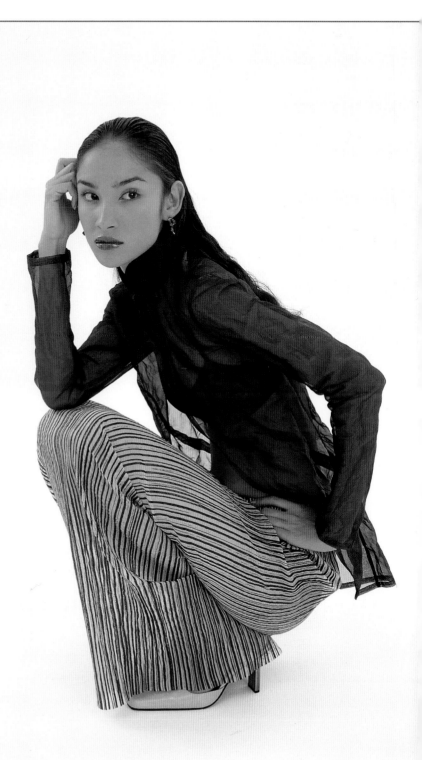

"Follow one navigational system and you always know where you are. Follow two and you're never sure."

I am a romantic, I embrace natural things. I don't necessarily like expensive things, but I like them to be tasteful. Hence I must continually cut through the veil between what I think the market needs and what it presently wants, then figure out how to fulfil them both. I want to recapture the East and the West and make it work. The West for its colour, for its look, its resources. The East for its textures, prints, patterns.

Local buyers are becoming prouder of our origins. We take more interest in native colours, prints, fabrics and everyday details, such as the many different ways to twist the sarong at the waist. I think of our neighbouring countries and all their rich resources and believe the ethnic look will make a strong comeback. If you work with colours in the right way, you can change the whole concept of ethnic.

Singapore's Asia New Tropical look uses more versatile elements for accessories, like wraps and carry-bags. It is a sensitivity to warmer cultures, warmer peoples, a feeling that the East-meets-West look isn't the only Asian identity that can be marketed internationally. Colours, style, prints and shopping experiences can all have both local and international appeal. Style is how we put these together, how we make it work and still stay simple. **"**

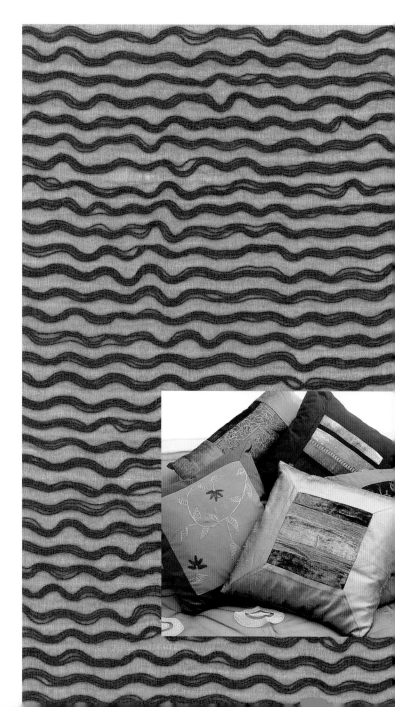

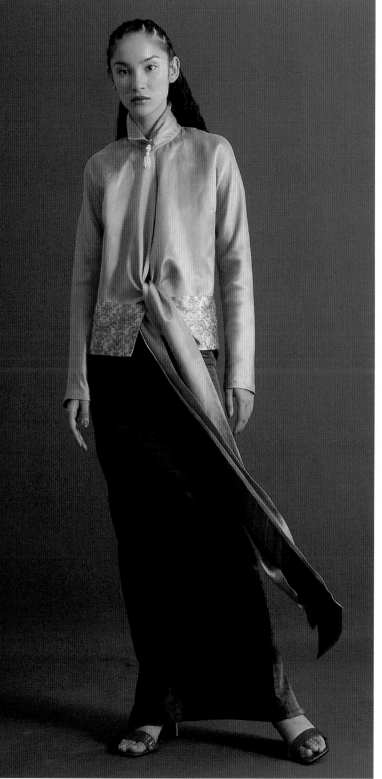

"I'm inspired first by fabric and colours. I will see an upholstery fabric and see possibilities for it – cushions, tablecloths, airplane carry-alls. You don't have to see fabric only as garments."

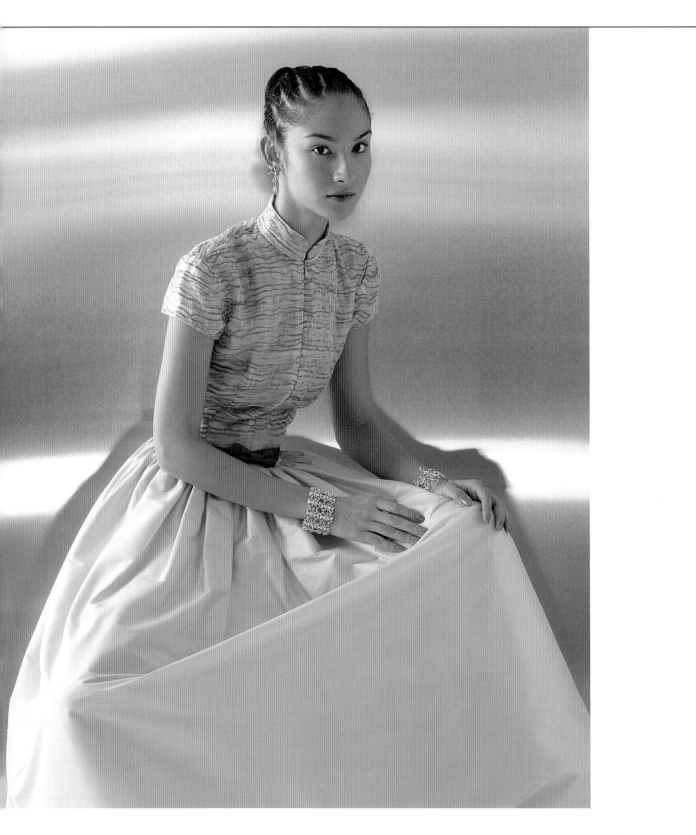

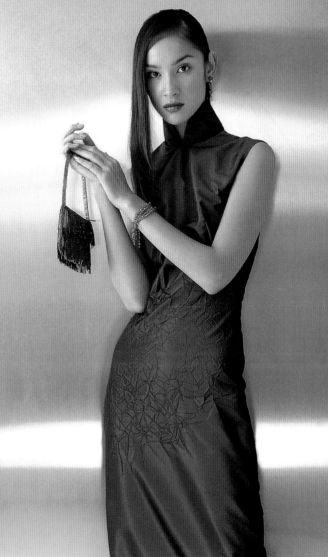

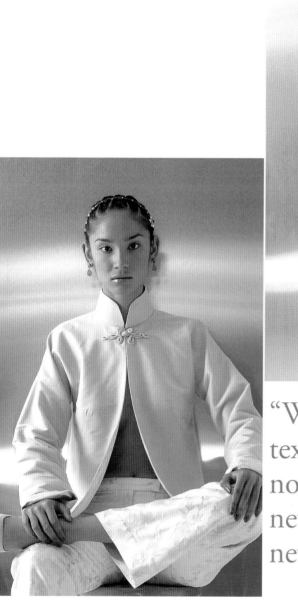

"With the richness of our
textiles resources, we can
now do much more with
new textures, new silhouettes,
new colours."

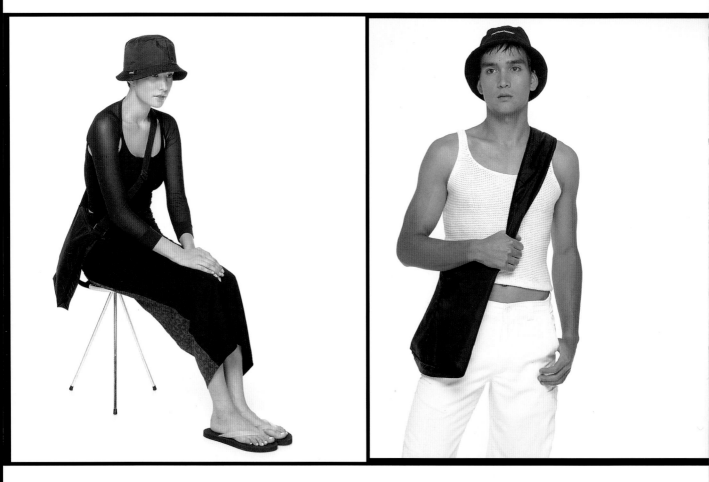

"Simplicity is always classic. It's always been there. Simplicity is sexy too. Maybe that's why it's so classic."

Peter Teo
Singapore

Singapore's minimalist fashion identity comes as a great surprise to those who think that because most of the population is Chinese, everyone runs around in cheongsams. Do Americans all wear stetsons and Frenchmen all wear berets?

Singaporeans are creating something called Asia New Tropical style. With its mix of old culture and new, of the natural and the technological, combined with a receptiveness to the interior of one's inner vision, Singapore's highly developed graphic sensitivity is attuned to local image and shape, complex exteriors and serene insides.

"The Singaporean design companies that do best are the ones that literally design weekly. That's how often people go shopping. This evolved from not having fresh stock from Europe for three to six months at a time. Once we started offering quicker collections, they soon became every two weeks because our customers liked it. Now it's every week.

This isn't easy. There are so many elements in putting a line together that it is hard to maintain a well-coordinated look while changing it all the time.

There's a lot going on in Singapore, but it is not centred on media and connections in the same way that it is in New York. In Singapore you don't need sales history or media history so much. The biggest Singaporean hang-ups are that artists don't deserve to get paid for what they love to do and that talking about one's ideas is considered self-advertising.

People here are rapidly becoming less conservative. This is happening so fast that it says something about the way taste is evolving on a mass scale. The more socially confined a Singaporean is, the less restrained their sexiness becomes in their clothing.

The public's taste in silhouette will probably stay clean, but it will be done in a totally different way. A big impact has come from stretch tailoring and stretch fabrics. A lot of design thinking in Singapore is watching the changing technology of fabric. "

Kevin Tsao Yao-Wen
Singapore

Until quite recently, 'style' had little meaning in Asia. The term only began to acquire significance when marketing experts started influencing business decisions. And, too, the idea that a garment can be hung on a wall like a painting is diametrically opposed to the Asian practice of packing one's finest garments safely away in wooden chests to prevent insects from ruining them. Consequently, the complex assembly and craft techniques of the American art-to-wear movement never really caught on in Asia.

Now, a few very young designers, such as Kevin Tsao and Cynthia Ng, are breaking away from the straitjacket of practicality to design garments which are pure form. Their experiments, however, are never likely to turn up in department stores, or, for that matter, in art galleries. Yet who is to say if the bold experimentalism now emerging in Singapore might not spawn geniuses of the calibre of Issey Miyake and Yohji Yamamoto in the future? We can only encourage youngsters like these, still in school and with little sense of boundary, to create as vividly as they can now and worry about their careers later. One day, Asia's nascent generation of designers will influence garment thinking far, far away.

"Fashion design is an art created through form, movement and communication. A clothing designer has more room to manoeuvre than in other art forms. We can express our feelings through silhouettes, colours, fabrics and, of course, through moments in motion.

Working with Singaporean designers is a superb opportunity to expand my horizons. A garment should create a dialogue, communicate with people. I never learned that idea in school. It is not something that can be taught. The saying, 'Learn to live, live to learn', is very real to me. Things are always changing, and changing rapidly. Thus, experimentation, research, reading and observation are important to me.

Being a fashion designer is a tough job. You really have to love your job, love every detail and process that you use. I have to create things that are new and that others have not thought of. It is vital to be curious about everything, to observe and be inspired by it.

Sometimes an inspiration comes to me when I am with people. I have always had a great interest in people. I learn an enormous amount from the way they behave. I cannot draw any new energy from within a design once I have completed it. To be in contact with other people's thinking gives me the impulse to create the next work of art. This helps me to stay fresh and energetic."

"Clothing is an art I express my feelings with, but not my egoism. Dialogue and communication between garment and wearer are very important; they reveal reality via movement."

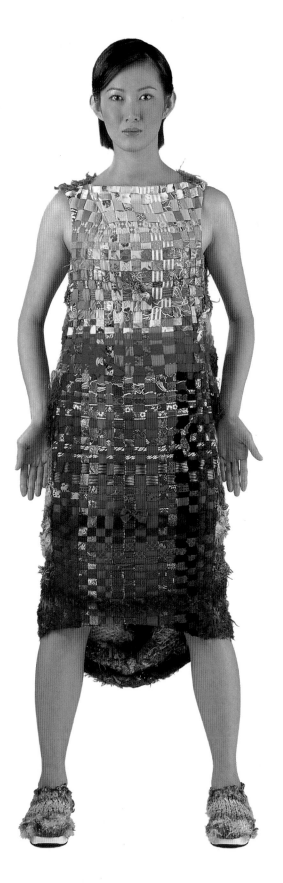

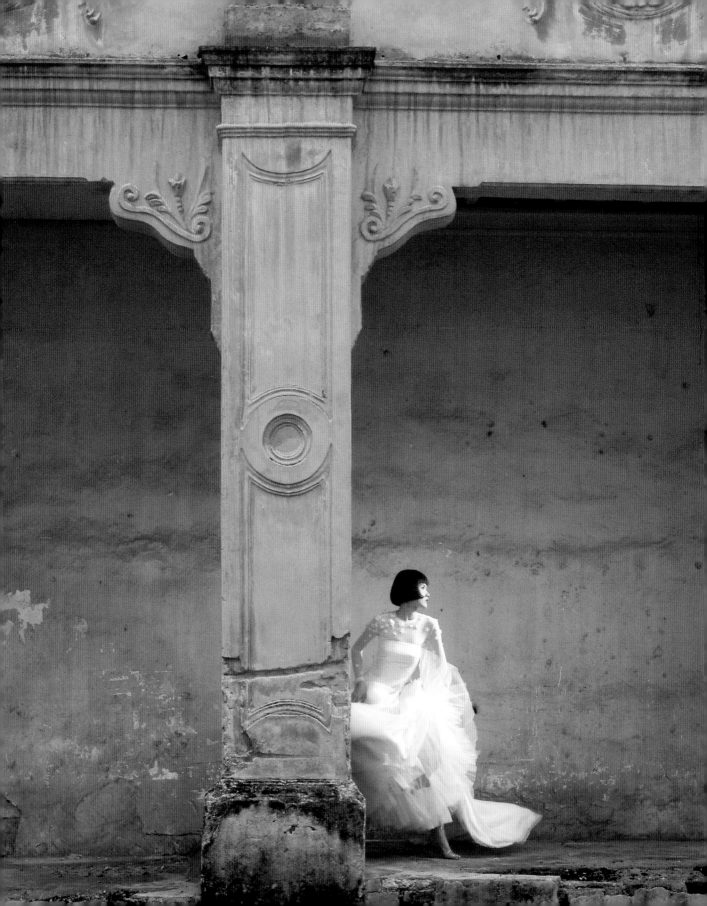

Tan Yoong
Singapore

"My clients know I specialize in exclusiveness. As a result, many young debutantes come to me seeking that extra-special birthday outfit or prom-night gown."

From the day Tan Yoong first opened his boutique in 1983, women flocked to buy his extravagant evening wear. His designs are ornamental, painstakingly embroidered, hand-appliquéd, quilted, beaded, pastelled. His signature is copious tiny embellishments on each outfit, often using vanishing craft techniques, ranging from subtle dyeing techniques to the making of the finest trim on knife-pleating. Surprisingly, his knowledge of beading, embroidery and three-dimensional appliqué is mostly self-taught. All it requires, so he says, is a good eye and a large dose of common sense.

His clients fall into two categories. The first is women who appreciate his use of pastels and handiwork in original design. The second is those with their own dress sense who ask him to translate their tastes into design creations. In turn, they recommend him to their daughters, sisters, relatives and friends.

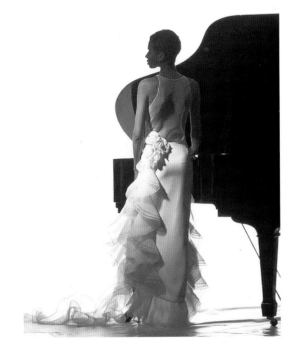

Malaysia
Beyond the Floral Ocean

Design by Rizalman

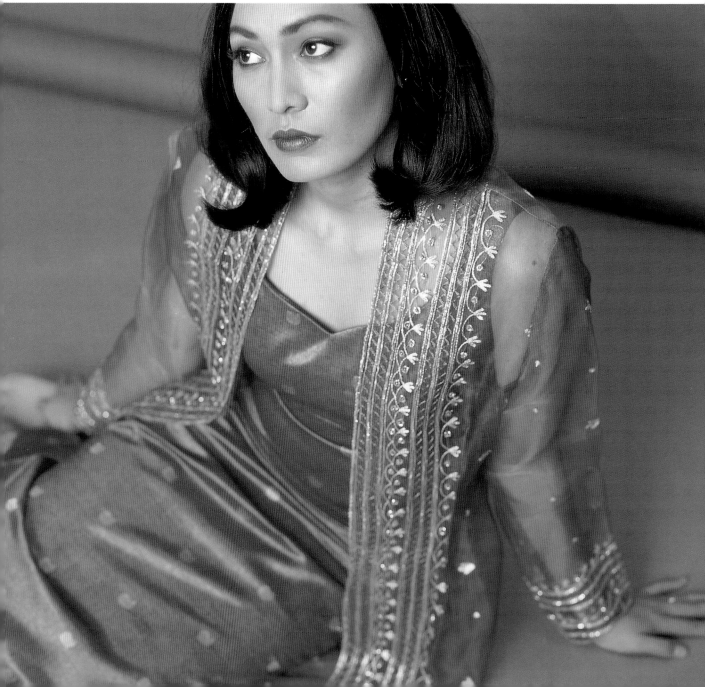

At five past five, Malaysia's office-wear women erupt from their workday routine. A rivulet here, a torrent there, fussy florals and saturated hues flow into the streets. From clerks to CEOs, Malaysian women dress as if they are birds on the Tree of Life.

Given Malaysia's bird-flecked flower-splashed forests, it is no surprise that vivid colour and pattern are the hallmark of its women's garment sensibility. The Malay dress named the *baju* comes in three forms. The traditional cloaky *kurung* is a tentlike sheath enveloping everything between the neck and the ankle. Its upscale sister, the sultanate and opulent *kebaya*, originated in the Portuguese waistcoat introduced via Malacca four hundred years ago. The *baju kedah,* a hip-length collarless half-Malay half-Thai jacket, first became popular as working women's garb in Malaysia's northern Kedah province and drifted south, gaining social status on the way.

By whatever origin, the baju uses surface decor to create a sense of bodylessness. It draws on every image and technique imaginable: embroidery, appliqué, brush painting, the calligraphy of imaginary alphabets, gold and silver threads, plum blossoms, flowers on trellises, rice sheaves, shells, swallow-tailed birds, butterflies, waves, interlocking geometries, medallions, hibiscuses and gentians and peonies, leaves, scrolls, basket weaves, fish scales, mountains, clouds, flowing water, chequerboards, circles. Such a tumultuous vocabulary easily ends in chaos, and often does. The streets of Kuala Lumpur resemble an aquarium moving in semi-unison to the swells and ebb of the stoplight sea.

According to Duarte Barbosa, a late fifteenth-century Portuguese writer, the Malay women of Malacca long had a custom of wearing a homespun sarong that reached from the shoulders to the ankle and was roughly twice the circumference of a pregnant woman. So why all the surplus cloth? Utility. Pure plain practicality. The extra length and width could be pulled over the whole body for sleeping, used as a bathing cloth, wound around the forehead as protection from the sun, turned into a makeshift cradle for infants, slung across the back and under one arm as a carry-all, and – when tired – turned into a hammock. Two bajus and you were prepared for just about anything.

It is a fashion adage that fixed functional form results in a great profusion of ornament. The baju kurung has never gone out of style because it did not originate with style in mind. Neither have the chador, tunic and muu-muu, all of which embody the same philosophy of form before style. They are as basic as garments can be, yet their ornamentation is the most diverse in the world of clothing art.

Today, as Asia meets Europe, Malaysia's designers are taking a new look at the traditional Malay baju and at the cheongsam introduced by the country's Chinese settlers. With one eye on the local market and the other on European imports, they find that there is a certain charming agreeableness to the idea of old wine served in new bottles.

The result is the development of a garment vocabulary that quotes the baju, cheongsam, kurta and salwar kameez right alongside Dior, Armani and Valentino. Malaysia's designers are fusing garment art with body art in a brand new and yet uniquely Malaysian way.

"People who come to Malaysia from abroad remark on how vivid the colours are here. I never think about them, but all of a sudden, there they are in my designs."

Sharifah Barakbah's batiks combine the sublime with the original in work that meanders, runs and wanders downwards and upwards and backwards, enveloping itself. It bursts out in brilliant colours, skids to a stop in fields of detail work, takes up forms, repeats them, breaks the repetitions, then ends them in graceful expanses of pure colour. Her tumultuous batiks are stylish because they are so painstakingly wrought and so completely trend-breaking. Yet in no way do they lose the sense for vivid colour and pattern at the heart of batik.

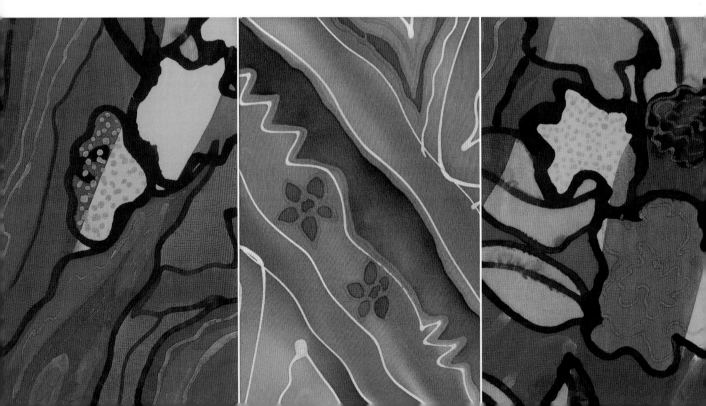

Sharifah Meheran Barakbah
Malaysia

"One day in primary school I decided I wanted to paint. So I walked into a store and asked the owner what to buy. The clerk was amused by this young customer, all by herself, wanting to buy paints but without the faintest idea of how to make green or brown out of red, yellow and blue.

I studied for four years, then got my own cottage and started making batik fabrics. At that time batik was not popular. It was still very traditional. People never messed with the motifs and colours, but I did.

I would take my things to boutiques and tell the owners I had an artisan's workshop where I did batiks. They would yawn, obviously having heard this before. Then I would open my bag and they would exclaim, 'This is batik!?' I got orders. They sold well. Somebody called it 'New Design' and I was suddenly taking trips to Singapore and places I had never dreamed of.

Ethnic art inspires my interest in both geometrics and fluid shapes: Sarawak's mingled curlicues, Native American designs, especially those of the Pueblos, who do marvellous things with ochre and dark yellow earth tones.

These traditional – but new traditional – designs appeal to younger Malaysians, to those who are changing our perception of style. Some say that international design is diluting our country's tastes. Maybe. But what I see more often is style-mixing between the different peoples of Malaysia and their respective traditional garments."

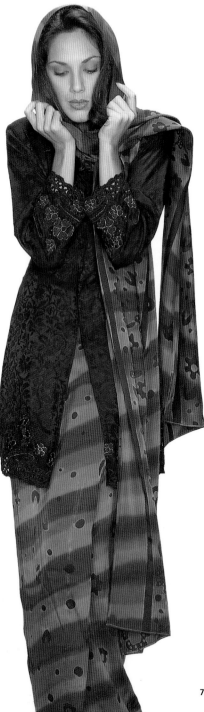

Bernard Chandran
Malaysia

Bernard Chandran is a mosaicist of fabrics, uniting colour and detail in garments so rich and regal they inhabit a god-kingdom of their own. His painstaking manufacturing process and the fineness of his details would come from the atelier of any Parisian couturier. Yet the designs on which he lays these could never be conceived in Paris. He has not tried to escape from European tradition; that would be simplistic. Instead, he has invented his own.

"I realized I wanted to do fashion design when I was fifteen. My father would allow me to go out on the town with friends. Usually we would go to the shopping centres to hang out. I loved the clothes, the noise, the people. Then one day I stopped by a fashion training school and was hooked.

From the day I started designing I wanted a glamorous look. When I first learned to cut for myself, I began to think of fashion as art rather than just clothing. When I cut the fabric myself, I find an idea and I come to know what I am making, instead of just dreaming it.

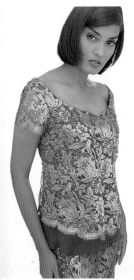
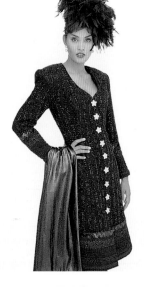

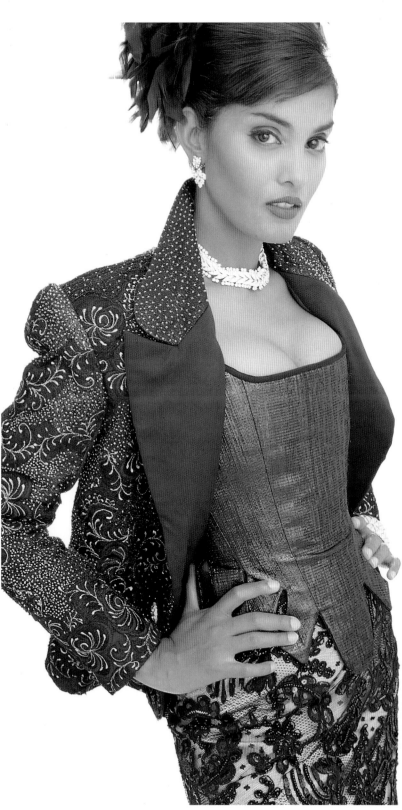

"After thousands and thousands of garments, I'm still only dressing up my dreams. Fashion is not the end. Art is not the end. Woman is the end."

"A woman must carry her clothes with character and refinement. That kind of woman is magical."

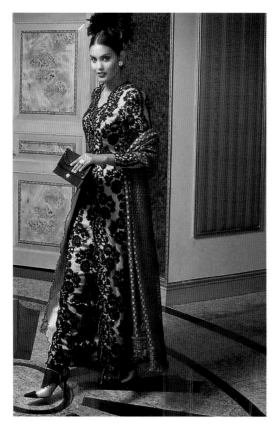

Sometimes I come up with a design as I drape. For every design, I produce three or four variations – different drapes, different cuts, a longer version, a shorter version. After seeing so many garments, I have by now an intuition of what will look good.

Usually I find a fabric, see that it is beautiful, but can't think of what to do with it immediately. Later inspiration comes. I'll be sitting down and I think, 'Oh, *that's* what it's supposed to be!'

Malaysia has a very complex culture, mixing elements of Malay, Indian and Chinese origin. We borrow from each other in interesting ways. The Malay people love beading and things that shine and look glamorous. Sometimes I give a Malay garment an Indian maharajah look to make it seem high fashion to local tastes. Other times, I'll mix different cultural themes together, like a Chinese cheongsam with an A-line look. Other times I'll take a clichéd idea like the satin stripe from the leg of a man's formal dinner trousers and translate it into women's wear by turning it into lace.

Clothing is just like art, like painting. Hanging in the closet a piece may look unimpressive, but when the person puts it on, it has to be art that they're wearing. "

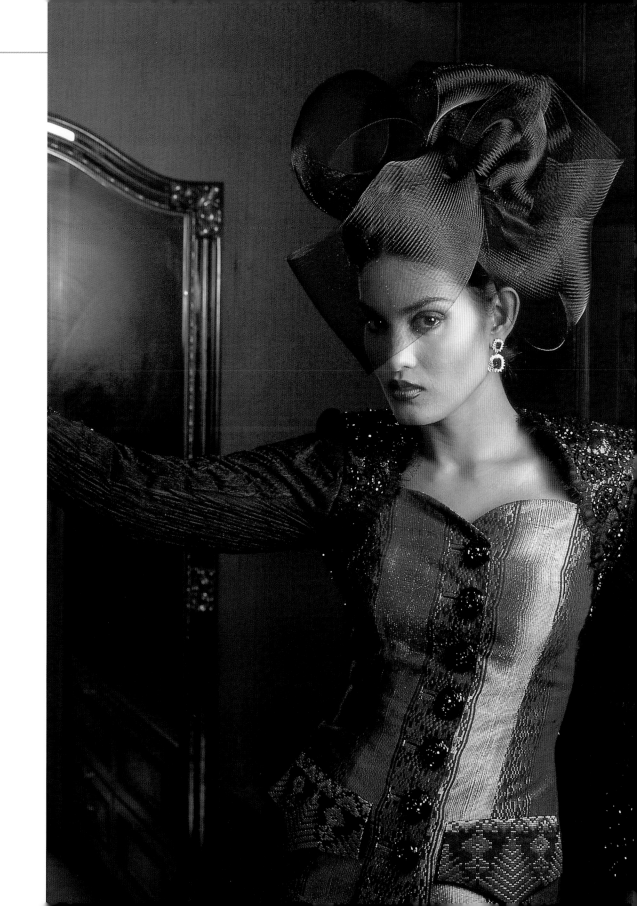

"Fashion is someone
communicating their
culture."

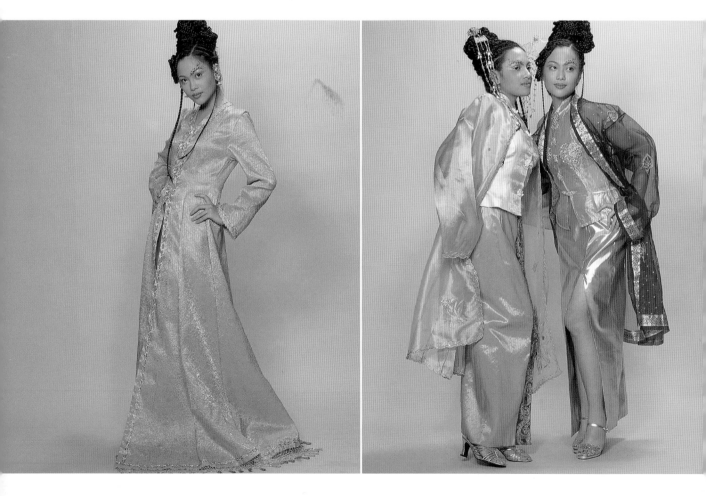

Bill Keith
Malaysia

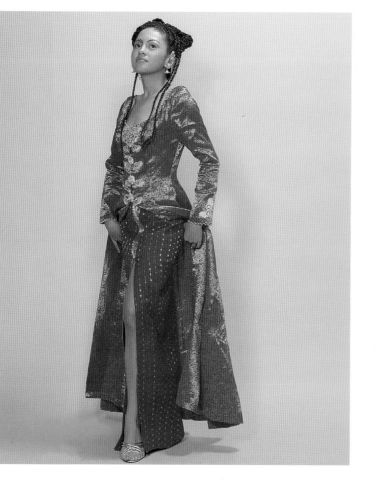

Bill Keith creates garments which, as he phrases it, 'transform the power of beauty into the power of self'. He is fascinated by the way that women have responded for centuries to certain design forms, such as the simple inner garment paired with the vividly hued outer garment. He begins his designs with the question 'What if?' and concludes with the fact that if wearer and garment compete, neither wins.

"I was a designer from before I could walk. On my first birthday, my parents followed the old Chinese custom of putting things on the floor – a screwdriver, hammer, spoon, scissors, book, umbrella and so on – believing that whatever I picked up would foretell my eventual career. I picked up a piece of fabric and a pair of scissors. My parents said, 'Oh, he's going to be a tailor.' At that time, the concept of fashion design did not exist in this part of the world.

Clothing is the art of the self. Your art-self is expressed in what you wear. When I see a person who sees the art in themselves, I see the identity, culture and values that lie beyond them. I watch and learn from them. The way a person walks inspires me to think of a fabric that will turn them into a totally different person.

Anything whose inner character is different attracts me. It is the motive of the fabric, its internal culture, that makes it unique. This is why traditional fabrics can be made into marvellously contemporary silhouettes.

My collections are rather traditional, in the sense of being typically Malay, in terms of depicting the country's many cultures, values, traditions and norms. I want to enhance their richness through the quality of the materials I use. I take a look at a swatch and ask what I can do with it; the identity of the fabric plays an important part. The swatch is already communicating whether it's Malay or Chinese or Indian. My first question is, 'How can I focus the eye on the part of the garment I most want people to see?' I do it in gestures with the fabric. Classic silhouettes are usually not very gestural, so I ask, 'What would I want more of, if I were in this?'

I try to create a masterpiece out of each piece. I don't call it fashion, it is art. **"**

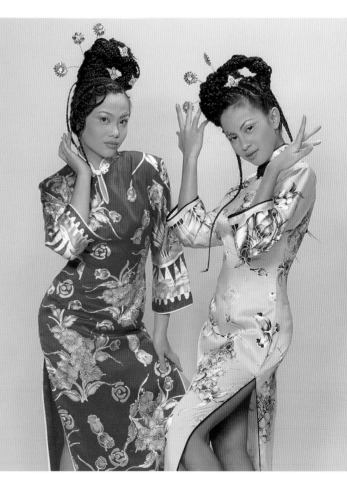

"I like to dress women as though they're from an indefinable place, a graceful, peaceful place, the place in their soul where they'd really like to be."

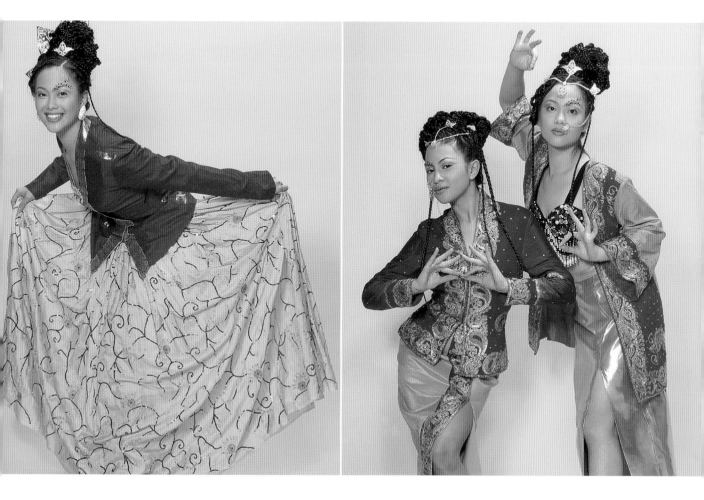

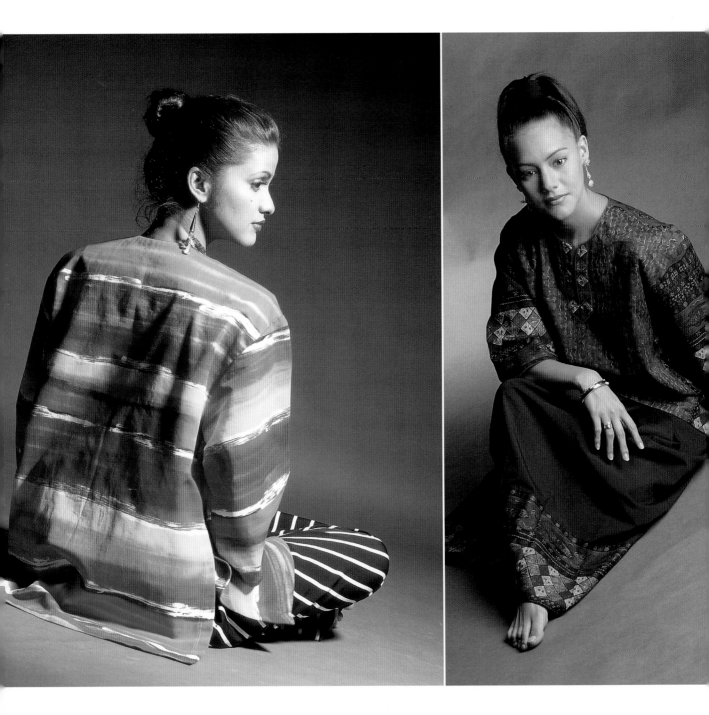

"My ideal garment is the essence of the traditional East – simple lines, comfortable, multi-functional, timeless. Women tell me they still can wear something they bought from me ten years ago and it works just as well as it did the first time."

Leung Thong Ping, or Pinky as she is known to her friends, reworks the cheongsam's body consciousness into silhouettes and surface designs you could easily wear at the Café de la Paix – in Shanghai! She knows that silhouette not only sculpts the wearer, but unites her clothes and her psyche. She translates the four elements of a woman's structure – shoulders/bust, waist, hips and legs – into a unique whole. In Pinky's hands, a woman is her own art form.

"My mother made clothes for the best-known women in Kuala Lumpur. Scraps of pretty fabric were always around. When I was about ten, I sewed a patchwork skirt from her remnants. Even then, the way I put together the colours was very different.

My first job was as a journalist. My sewing was a weekend hobby, but my unusual wardrobe got a lot of attention. My earliest creation was a tangerine batik sarong with dark green and brown patterns. A piece of

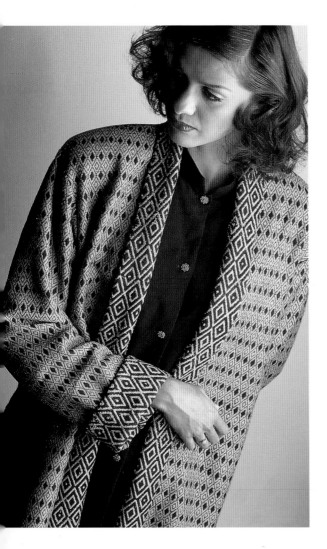

border for the yoke stretched snugly across the chest much like a Balinese dancer's costume. It was both beautiful and functional. You could go out in it, sleep in it, expect a baby in it.

Fashion design is a limited experience on a daily basis – you are more in contact with fabric, cutters, sewers and marketers than anyone else. My academic rather than fashion-oriented training and my subsequent work experience with the newspaper exposed me to a world of fashion thinking much more than if I had gone to a design school.

Hence I don't much go by theory. I know instinctively what works and what doesn't. Most often I am inspired by women on the street. They don't wear design, they are design. Wildly gorgeous and uncontrolled combinations of colours and forms flash by. I get an idea and intuitively know exactly which fabrics will work best with it. The part of the garment that's nearest the face gets looked at the most, so I put a lot of thought into the treatment of collars, necklines and sleeves. To make an outfit interesting, I do not always use predictable linings in plain colours; mine are often small patterned prints.**"**

"Traditional garments are the epitome of economic design – they're mostly just squares and oblongs fitted together. The sarong is so popular because it is a piece of art. I could work wonders within the confines of the sarong, with the textures, patterns and unusual colours you can introduce into one."

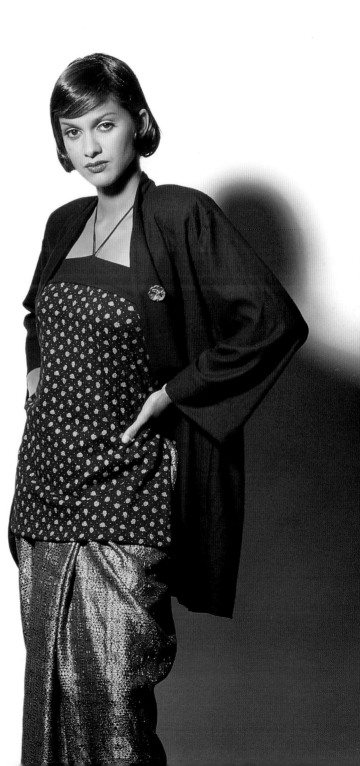

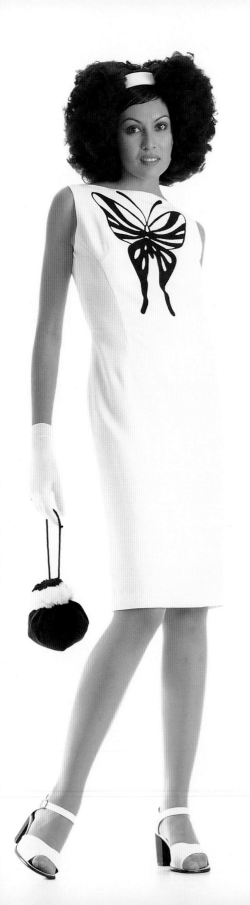

Carven Ong
Malaysia

Carven Ong's designs convey the multiplicity of the self through the simplicity of shape. He implies a woman of complexity by reducing everything she wears to its simplest surface self. He is so scrupulous with detail that his designs approach pure form. The body is its own architecture. The eye is confronted with the psychological implications of a single unadorned shape. The absence of any other relationship is like a person dancing brilliantly yet alone in a crowd.

"I was about seven when I first began to draw. I loved taking blank paper and drawing the clothes women wore. My teachers saw this and encouraged me. I became known as Carven Who Likes To Draw.

Aged about seventeen or so, I would watch TV and movies, pretending to design for the singers and the stars. I was interested in what they wore and tried to duplicate it myself.

My parents weren't thrilled about the idea of me taking a career in fashion. They thought it wasn't a line of work suited for a man. But since I was so keen on it, they let me.

"I will be doing more and more black and white, emphasizing the white."

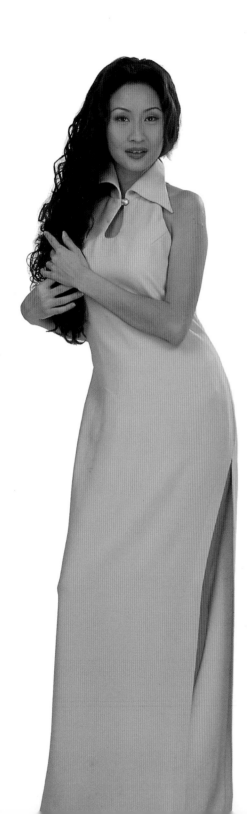

"I prefer solid colours because they don't date so quickly."

I started my business after I won first prize in a contest in Kuala Lumpur. A lot of students wanted me to start my own school. I began with only seven students. Others heard and came. I taught fashion illustration using marker pens. A lot of schools wouldn't touch the things I did.

In Malaysia it takes time for trends to take hold and it is difficult to introduce new designs to the average buyer. Overseas designers design for shows, but we have to design for customers. So my garments have to say something special. That's why I have two lines: one for business and one for shows.

My signature is softer edges and silhouettes and I use romantic, elegant fabrics like chiffon. I sometimes like the Chinese style: their colours and embroidery and the cheongsam. My favourite designers are Lagerfeld, Chanel and Yves Saint Laurent.

I do office wear because it varies relatively little. All my work is for women. I am planning a teenage line, but haven't decided on a label, but I analyse the market as being for fifteen- to twenty-one-year-olds. **"**

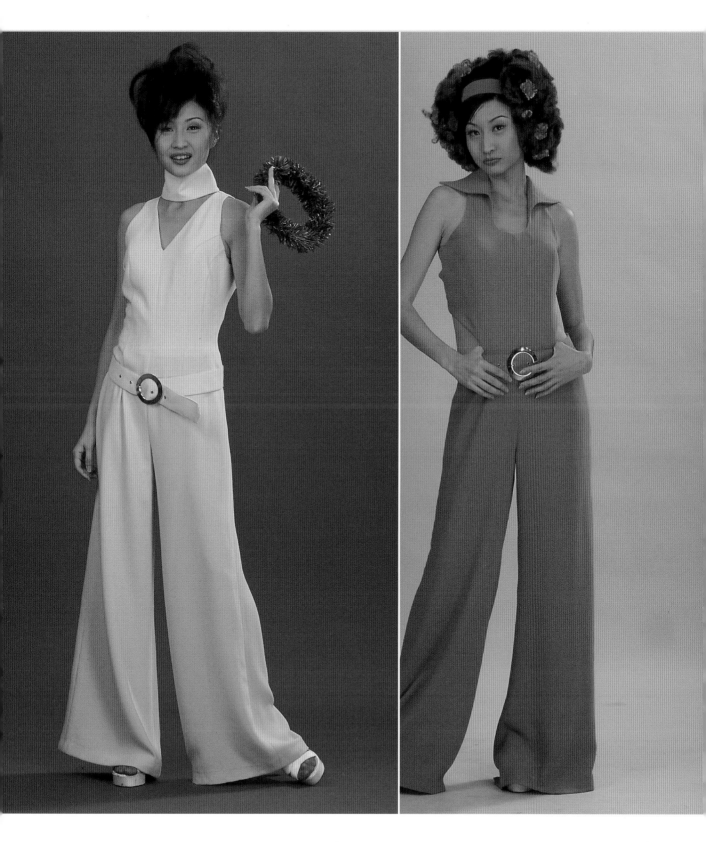

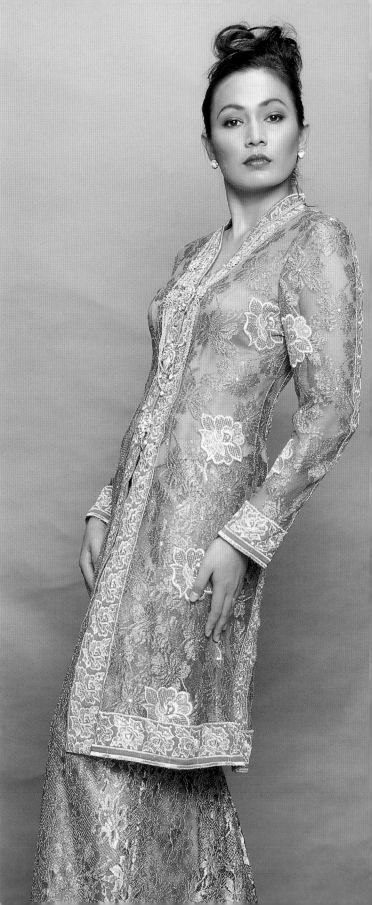

Rizalman
Malaysia

How can you live in Malaysia and not say so!

"I grew up in Georgetown, Penang Island. Nothing in my childhood attracted me to fashion, but I loved to draw using pencils and watercolours. When it was time for technical training, I thought about graphics, but at the time too many people seemed to be going into it. Ceramics had no future. So fashion was the choice and I just jumped into it. The course took three years. I was particularly interested in handling fabrics and won a competition in which I was given a few metres of fabric and a mannequin and told to create an evening gown.

I concentrate on the Malay baju kebaya and baju kurung for my basic designs. I then add contemporary ideas, particularly ideas about simplicity. I am attracted to traditional Malay styles in part because so many of our designers are now embracing foreign silhouettes and ideas. That's fine, but I am a Malay and I have my own cultural heritage

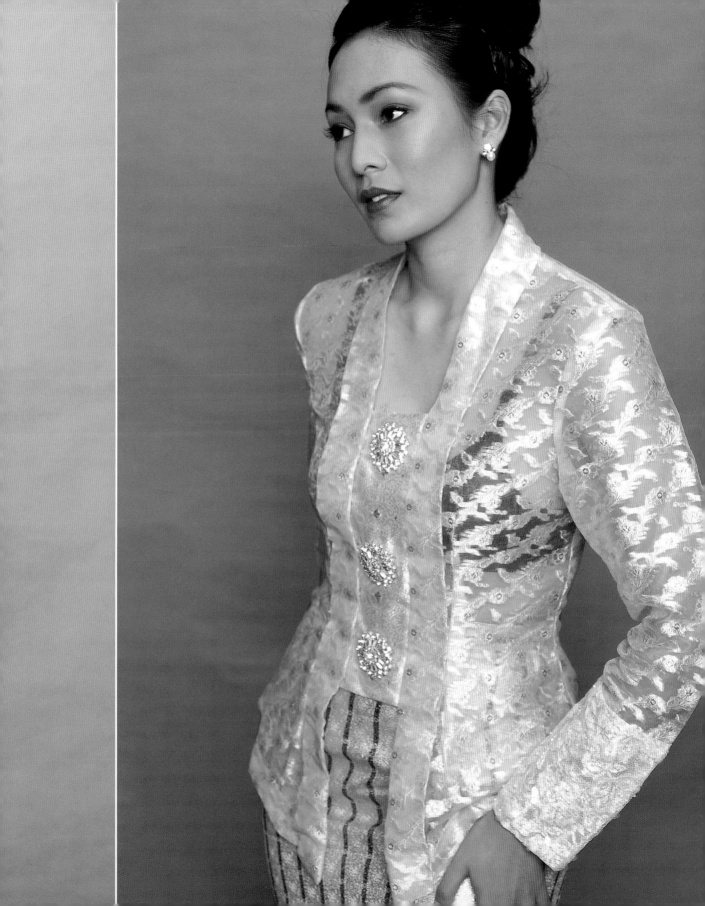

"A garment has an internal integrity which sets its own limits. If you try to impose your own ideas on that integrity, the results can be awful."

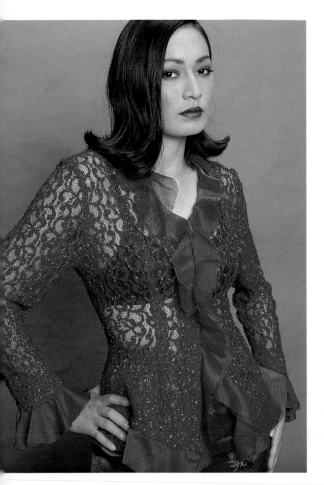

that I want to show the world. We can offer the West some original ideas, especially with cut and silhouette. Our sensibility with regard to a woman's nature is that her strength and essence are tempered by her vulnerability. That's why the shawl and the *tudong* head scarf are so indicative of the culture here.

As with a lot of designers, it is the fabric that inspires me. I love warm pastels, although some traditional combinations use bright or shocking colours well. For example, the green of Islam looks good with the yellow of the sultans.

I shall probably not go into commercial production. In Malaysia one can profit more quickly – though less handsomely – with personal clothes than by cranking out thousands and thousands of mass-produced garments. Most Malaysians prefer made-to-order rather than ready-to-wear, but the time pressures of city life are changing their attitudes. **"**

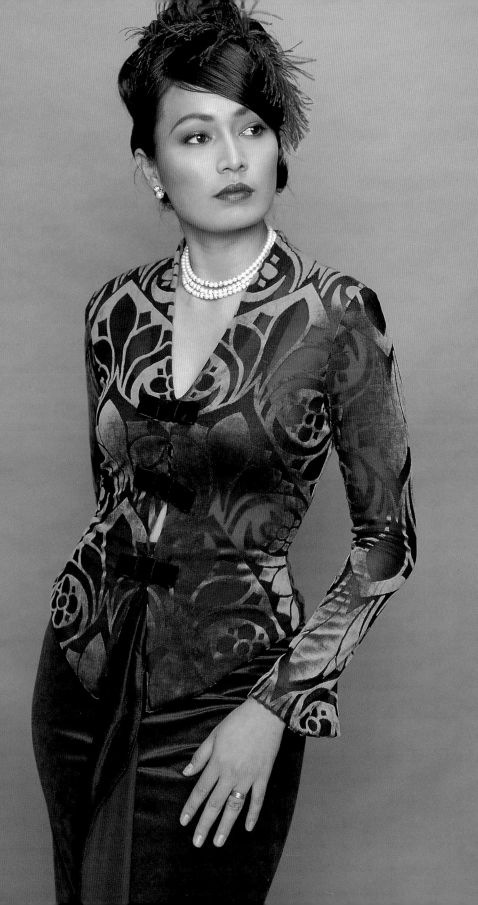

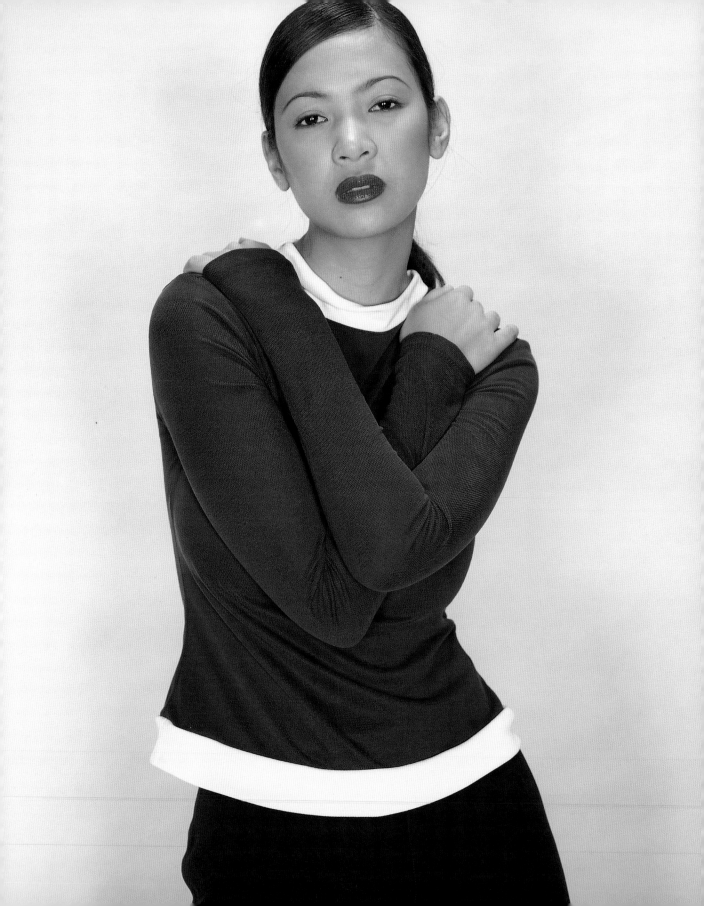

Edmund Ser
Malaysia

Edmund Ser marries garment and city in such a way as to create a modern tribal feel. His office and after-five wear look beyond decorative sensations, such as colour and cut, into the relationship between men and women and their surroundings. His work is what happens to theatre when you take away the stage: the play becomes the audience.

"Clothes designing – as distinct from tailoring – was a new idea in Malaysia in the 1980s when I got started. The people who had money weren't spending it on fashion. Today things are different. A lot of people are looking for someone not only to supply them but also to guide them. I must give customers a product that everyone knows is from Malaysia.

In this part of the world we don't have seasons. We redesign our women's line every week with new items, new fabrics. Our gentlemen's line changes every two weeks. With colours we're restricted pretty much to availability, but our fabrics and designs change literally every week. Our customers expect to walk in and see something new every Saturday – that's the nature of shopping here. I have to know their tastes, their mentality, their reactions, their feelings, the changes they will want. Pleasing people is the key to pleasing yourself.

We cut each design in four sizes and as many colours as are available – three, four, ten. We make five pieces in each colour and each design. We ship one design per outlet to our five outlets. That way people can be sure they get a unique item. Once a design is finished, we don't go back to it. And once a bolt of fabric is finished, we don't go back to that either."

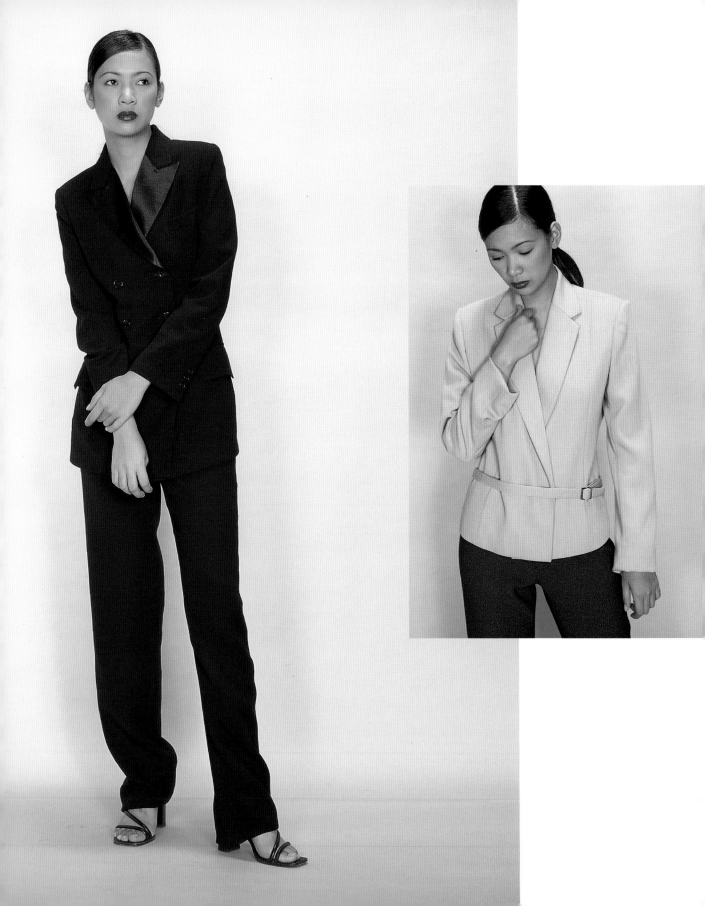

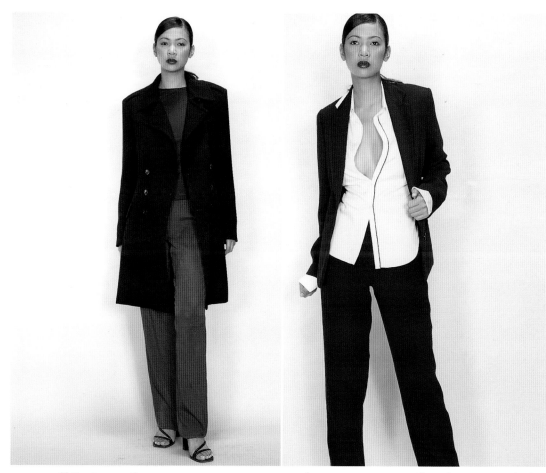

"My clients are mostly young fashionable people – key people in new, energetic businesses. They don't particularly like the hard look and feel of traditionally tailored garments and fabrics."

Thailand
Art Directing the Self

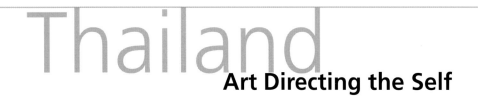

Fabric by Nagara

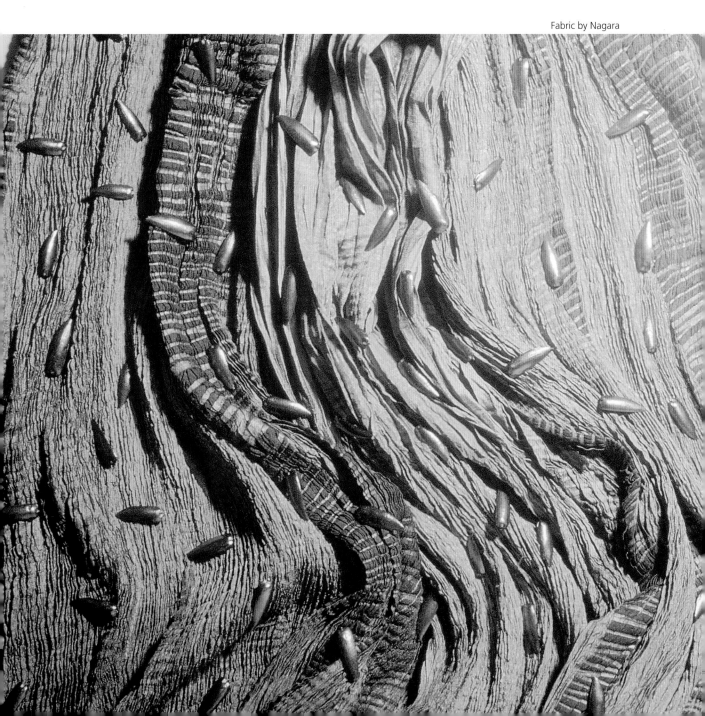

The overriding quality of Thai design is its Buddhist philosophy of not too much and not too little. Even though many Thais are not that familiar with Buddhism's doctrines, they certainly know the Middle Way. For Thai women, this is in part a merging of the imported and the local. They have their strong ethnic and cultural identity, but they are also influenced by foreign styles and ideas.

Thailand's largest, yet least influential, category of clothes buyers is called 'the middle-class young consumer group' by Asian marketers and 'Missy' in the West. The age bracket is much broader than in the West: from thirteen to twenty. The reason for such a wide span is that, in relation to age, silhouette changes little among younger Thai women. Their body shape remains girlish four to five years longer than with the Western Missy. Since shapeliness is an intense preoccupation for those who lack it, Asian Missies go for a spray-painted viscose look.

The Thai Missy adores Western-brand casual wear. Brand power is important because most young Thai women have only a nascent idea of personal taste, particularly in the cities where almost everything of the old Thai culture has been consigned to the tour-bus set.

All this is a terrible drain on a father's Visa card. Missies and their Cubbie boyfriends (named after the 50cc Honda Cub, the only transportation they can afford) have no incomes of their own and the brands they crave are expensive. The 1997 economic collapse devastated the budgets of a large percentage of the middle class, so keeping up with the Ruksajits is a lot harder than it used to be.

Most Thai women begin to develop their own taste sensibility around twenty to twenty-five. This is the age when they first become aware of the discourse between the fantasist that is the designer and the critic that is the body. It is an age bracket where fashion identity is torn between simplicity in style and decoration, on one hand, and colourful, costumey complexities on the other. Many women simply buy both.

Before the economic crisis, these women looked to the West – largely via glossy women's magazines – for their ideas and sensibilities. It is hard to tell if they were first attracted to Western fashion because of the simplicity of the designs or because it was simply 'in' to buy imported. Now that people have become intensely price-conscious, it has led inevitably to simpler silhouettes and darker, more neutral colours that can survive for longer between dry-cleanings.

High-income career women and the social elite go for classic styles with simple colours and natural neutrals. These are the women who put *hauteur* into haute couture. They have an unerring sense of balance combined with a daring appetite for form and for the fluidity that defines the shapely and the energetic from the plain. It is here where you find those luscious extravagances of tulle and organza, chiffon and taffeta, silk and satin. It is rare for them to use only two colours. Their social status places them at the junction between past and present, yet they are committed to the conscious hand of the designer's art in a world as ethereal as wealthy women. Ancient icons on fluid modernity.

Nagara

Nagara's design shows are dramas in which garments play an important, but not dominant, part. He integrates themes that continuously well up inside Thai people: the garments themselves, snatches of music, dreams, traditional body motions like those of the dance or court ritual, the mix between costume and story. You might think from this wild combination of elements that somehow the reason for the garment – the woman who will wear his clothes – is forgotten.

Not so. She is the queen of the event. She sees herself not merely as part of the drama, she *is* the drama.

"I came to fashion design via interior design. My father wanted me to be an architect, but I started batik painting as a hobby. This in turn led me to the creation and printing of textiles. Then I studied traditional Japanese dyeing and weaving with a master of age-old techniques at Kameoka in Kyoto.

Today I am the only Thai fashion designer who makes his own fabrics. They are hand-woven at Karat in eastern Thailand. I do this partly to be in complete control of my work, but, more importantly, so I am not dependent on the market. Silk weaving has a long history of technological development in Thailand and we are extremely lucky that Her Highness Queen Sirikit strongly supports the Thai textiles weaving community by wearing Thai garments on so many occasions. Her generous financial support is invaluable to the schools that keep our tradition alive.

In my work room on the northern outskirts of Bangkok, I have a special weaving and textile laboratory set up to experiment with new effects and the techniques needed to achieve them.

When I create a design for a particular piece of silk, the earliest stage is sifting through impressions of shape and texture from some often quite mundane things: wood grain, concrete, the time of year, street scenes, the basic elements, shapes and colours that flash before my eyes. I work quite a bit with Thai *ikats* in which the colour is woven in (and sometimes even dyed directly on) the loom."

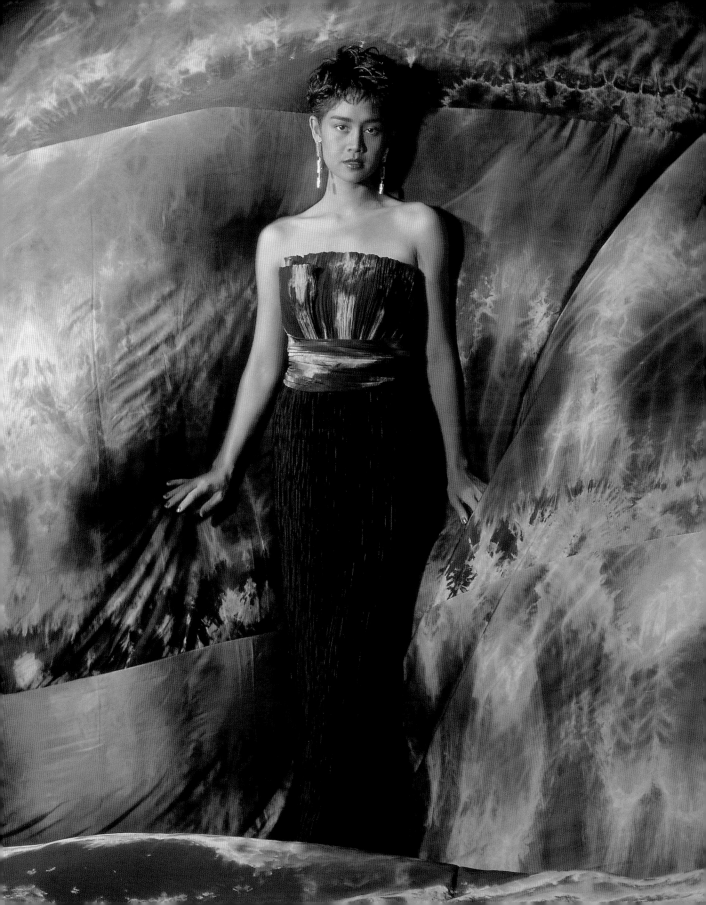

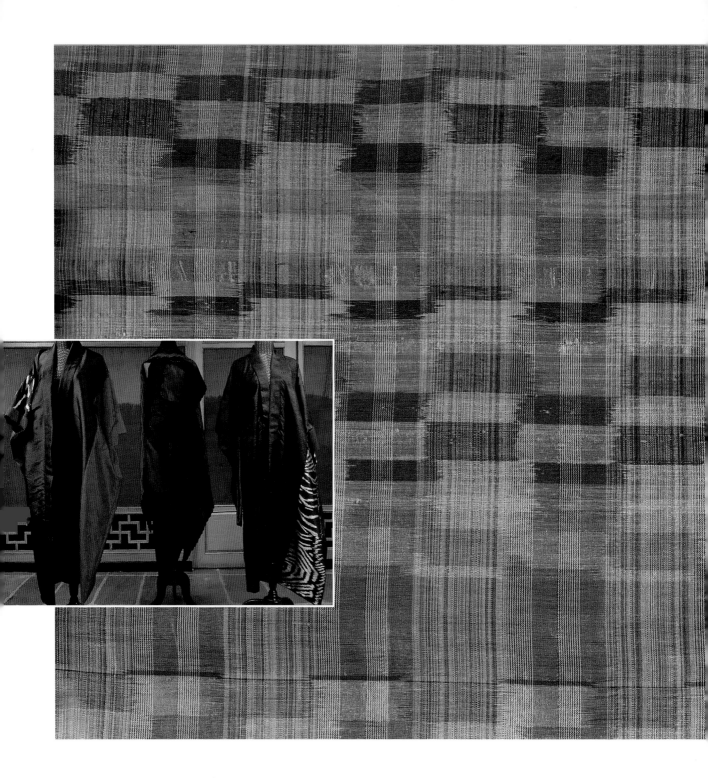

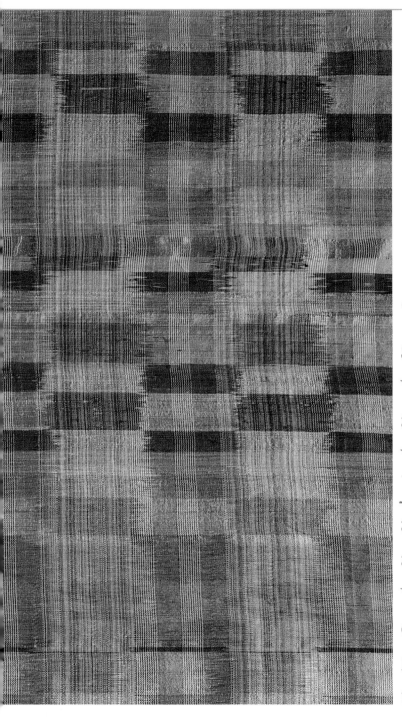

"All my designs start off in some way with Thai tradition and culture, laced with a touch of Japanese, Chinese, and Indian garment art. I make regular visits to all these countries to keep myself aware of textile developments and availability there."

Sahasab Pinprachasan
Thailand

Establishing yourself in Thailand today is very different from doing so several years ago, when there were few designers and an extremely large clientele. That, plus the familiarity many upper-class Asians had with Europe from their student or business travel, influenced many Asians to turn to European designers.

Now, most Asians are spending less and therefore taking a second look at their own design communities. They are finding that local quality is just as good and the prices considerably lower.

Sahasab Pinprachasan entered the public arena at the 1999 Hong Kong Young Designers Show. He is still largely unknown abroad and, indeed, within Thailand itself. He is included in this book precisely because of his youth in the profession. The photograph and the sketches of his work shown here give some idea of the slender beginnings of almost every designer in this book. Yet you can tell from the many ways he can handle a single theme that he has the makings of a fine designer. Indeed, his ability to derive so many variations from a few simple givens puts him more in the category of Singaporean than Thai designers.

"When customers comes to see me, I ask what they want – office wear, a cocktail party dress, after-five, evening wear. I do a few sketches, show the kind of fabrics I think will be right. Once the basic design is done, I modify and expand it with different manifestations of the same theme, varying placements and the structural composition. If the customer wants a complex garment, I elaborate it carefully, sketch by sketch with the customer advising me.

My designs go from simple to quite complicated, depending on the occasion. My winter collections are inspired by simplicity, warmth and the fact that many of my buyers travel internationally in winter.

Our Thai fables and legends make us different from the rest of Asia. We use more techniques and patterns from the past than elsewhere, except perhaps for Indonesian designers. Old costume has a huge effect on our sensitivities.

Beyond clothing, I am most inspired by architecture. I translate the slenderness of a standing column of an old Greek temple into a slender dress rising high above the waist; the capital becomes a wrap around the shoulders that extends part-way down the arms. The message I want to convey is that the woman is a column of strength, surmounted by a strong yet delicate beauty."

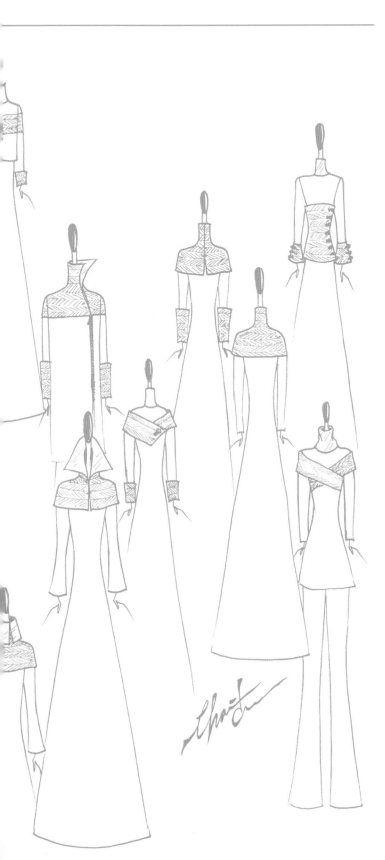

"I want to make the woman who wears my clothes beautiful and elegant. My dress must be suitable for her occasion, not mine."

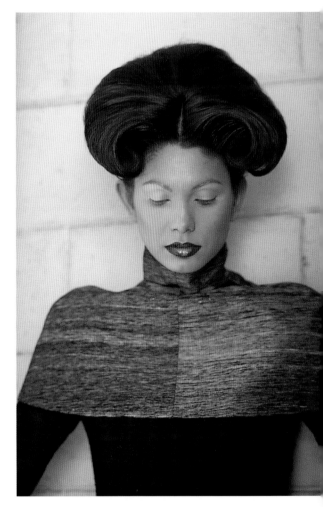

The Philippines

Weddings and Opulence

Design by Inno Sotto

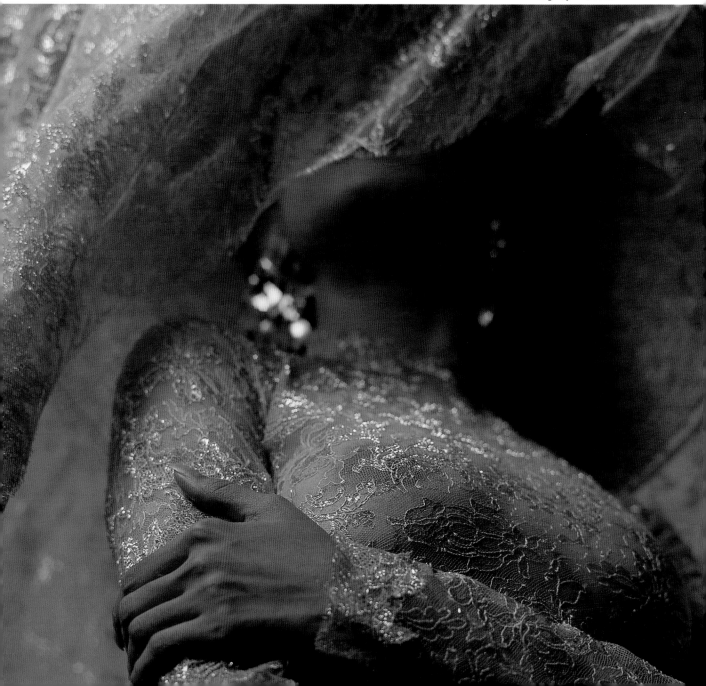

The Philippine doyen of haute couture, Inno Sotto, puts it perfectly: 'A Filipina is a study in event management. Her wedding is where she first sets her own standards. Other parts of the world have the grand ball, the grand entrance, the grand promenades, the grand opera. We have weddings.'

In the Philippines, the place to assert the primacy of the self is the wedding. Nothing is left to chance. A big wedding starts with the top names in Philippine fashion. Mothers want strength of vision and integrity of design. They also want an event that no one will forget.

'Fashion is driven by show', Inno believes, 'Filipinas are independent, extravagant, indulgingly courted and wooed, and dramatic about it. "If you want me to commit to you, I will. Lastingly. But my name must be in the starring role." For a man to be unfaithful is unforgivable. "It was your idea to woo me, so how can you now do this?"'

Drama is the essence of the Filipina. When she was First Lady, Imelda Marcos paid her designers in plain brown envelopes – manila, of course. Clothes for the sumptuously prosperous woman owe their success to silhouette. The Filipina is like a television production; she is composed of many well-edited shots. Her dress is designed to make her every movement a focus of action, give form to her every curve, put meaning into her every gesture, bring colour and life into her every event.

The fashion designer designs the entire wedding down to the last detail, including the gowns for the bridesmaids, what the ushers wear at the church, the hotel reception, even the table settings. Fashion is art direction.

In some parts of the world, women only appear in public after six in the evening. Their dress designers only have to create gowns. Not so in the Philippines. Filipinas, far more than other women in Asia, are active in the fields of business and charity work. Their designers have to create day wear, cocktail dresses, wedding gowns and evening wear. All custom-designed. A qualified Manila designer must produce at least eight hundred original creations a year. A client going on holiday or on a cruise will order twenty-five to forty outfits and won't tolerate repetition or knock-offs. It is the most demanding couture hothouse in the world.

'It takes ten years to acquire that kind of range', philosophizes Inno Sotto. 'The Philippine fashion landscape is littered with what we call the "Bogdanovich/Cimino Effect", one-hit wonders with one or two sensational seasons and then nobody hears about them any more. They run out of steam. They begin to quote themselves. That's the end.'

The successful designer cannot ignore criticism, nor can he or she succumb to praise. It is not design for design's sake. It is design that makes sense of the tumultuous world of Philippine wealth.

Cesar Gaupo
The Philippines

Cesar Gaupo is the Philippines' high priest of 'unicasional' fashion – free-flowing carefree clothing that also looks good at glamorous functions. High-spirited without aiming at the youth market, alluring without being Missy. His silhouettes articulate Manilan sensibilities in the same way that floral oceans say 'Kuala Lumpur' or Asia New Tropical says 'Singapore'. His emphasis is on ready-mades that hold their shape without hours of ironing. His garments can be worn anywhere and give Filipinas a stylish yet hometown-girl look.

"I became interested in clothes when one of my secondary school teachers saw my drawings and told me, 'You should buy some fashion magazines and try to copy those.' In professional illustrations, I saw how different approaches to life could be expressed so clearly in lines and colours. At first I thought fashion design was about capturing the essence of someone. I didn't yet know about fabrics, about construction. Straight after high school, I asked myself, 'Why go to college?' I just started designing and never stopped.

I learned the crafts of proportion, construction, execution and so on. I did my first show in the early 1970s and was soon 'discovered' by a client who suggested that I do ready-to-wear instead of made-to-order. I replied that I didn't have the experience, that I didn't know merchandising. He said I could learn from him.

So I did. I started with display windows, then went on to promotions, publicity, advertising campaigns, things like that. The upshot was that I opened my own boutiques within the chain of Shoe Mart department stores.

When I begin a design, I look for the fabric first. Something that is good for short skirts or sleeves won't work full length. Once I've found the right fabric, I know exactly what to do.

Texture, weave, drape and feel are all elements of a good design. But it is the *motive* of the fabric that attracts me. Inner character of any kind fascinates me, whether it is in architecture, nature, a gold fabric with eyelets, the architecture of a temple, a woman, a lily, a lotus. I like to preserve nature in everything I do.

For me the first expression of an idea is always the right one. I don't turn left, I don't turn right. If I change something, I inevitably end up going back to the original. I know I'm right when people see the idea and say, 'Wow! What a LOOK!' If an idea doesn't work the first time, it never will."

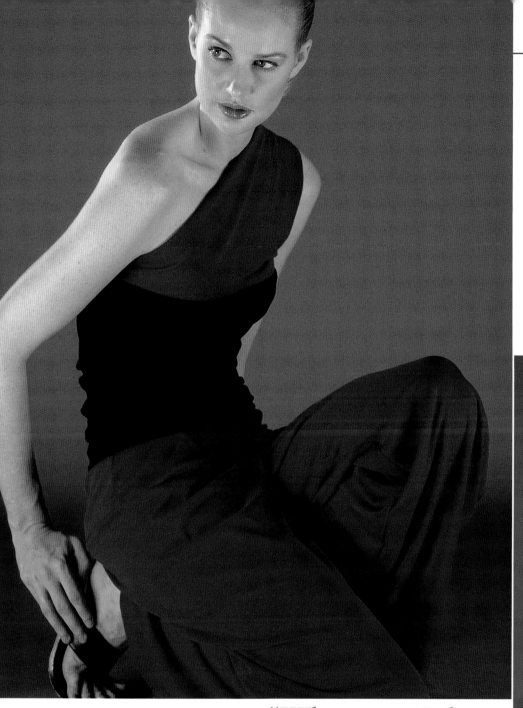

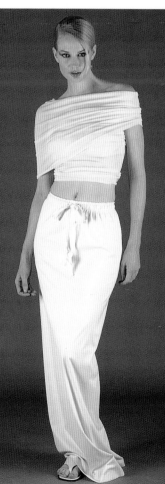

"Whomever I dress,
I am a little part of them.
They are a little part of me."

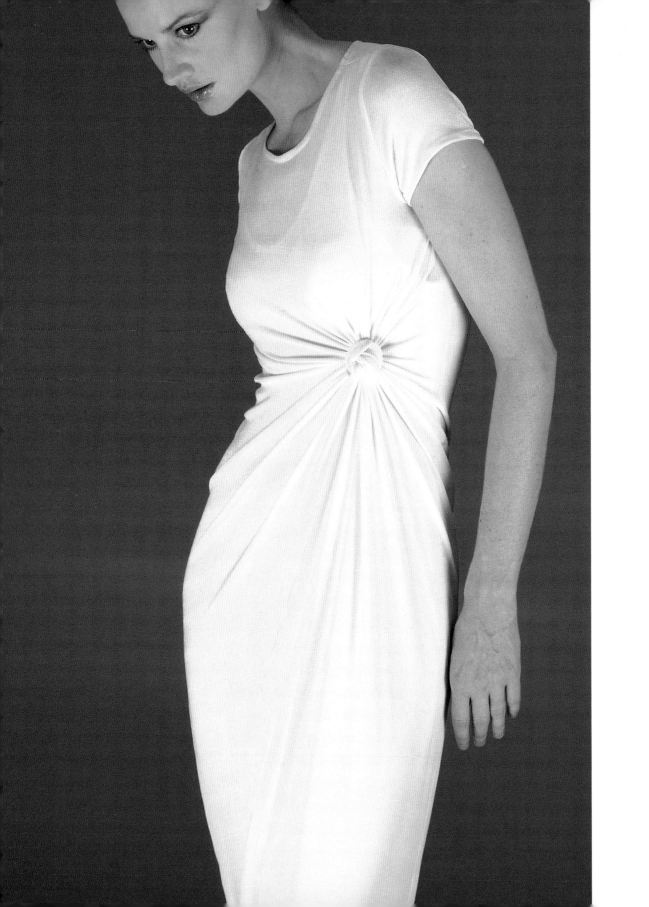

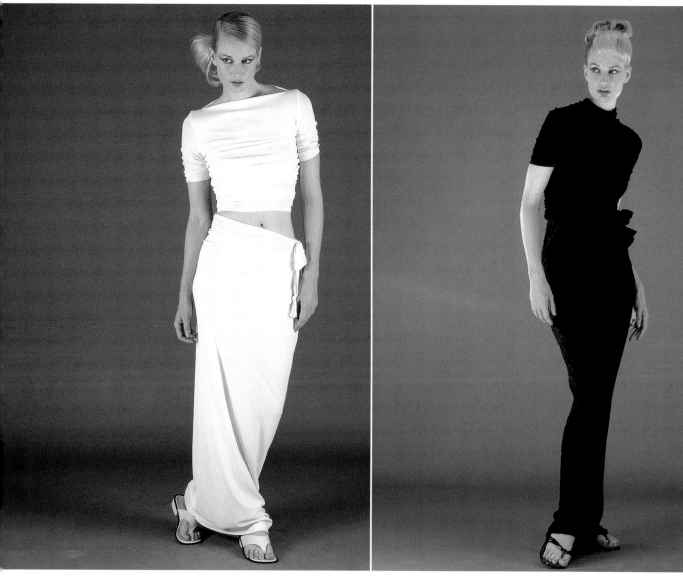

"I'm inspired by a woman who looks different from the others. The way she moves. The way she talks. Her sensibilities and her attitudes. The way she is with other people. The way she looks good, even when doing nothing. The way she is so languid, so cool. The way her facial expressions are so soft. When I see a woman like that, there's this sudden rush of creativity."

"When I see a woman who dresses herself as she really is, I see what she values beyond herself. Many people dress with attitude because they think attitude is the ultimate success. It isn't. The art of success is the art of self."

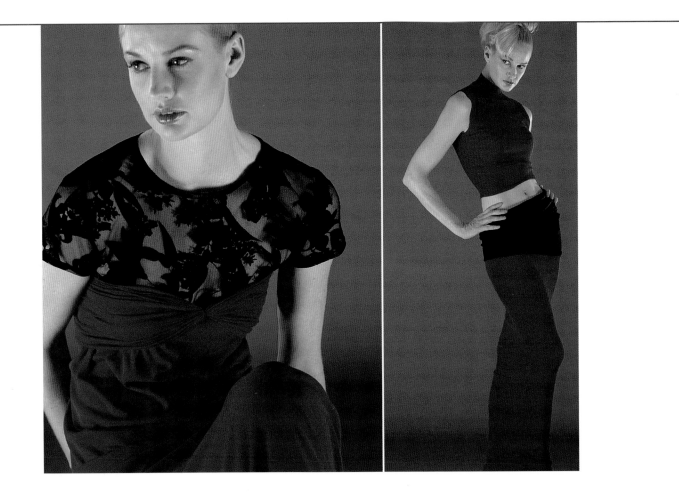

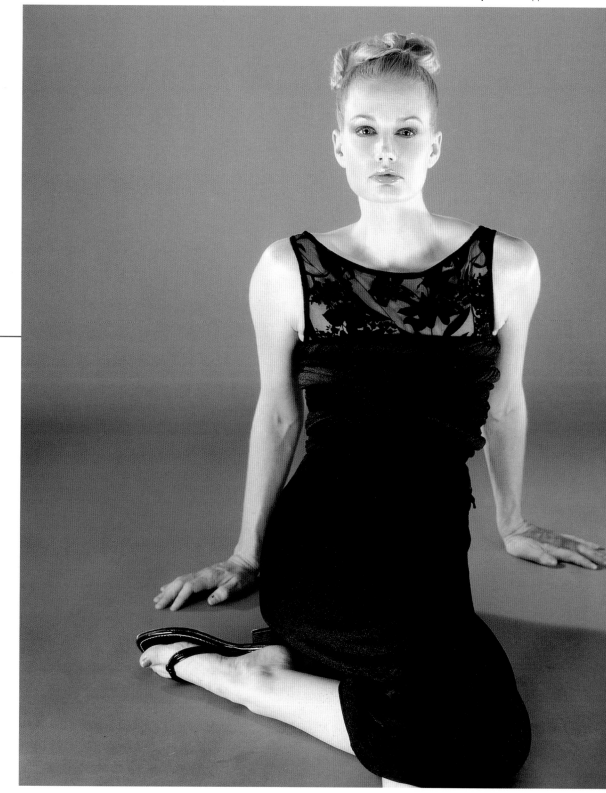

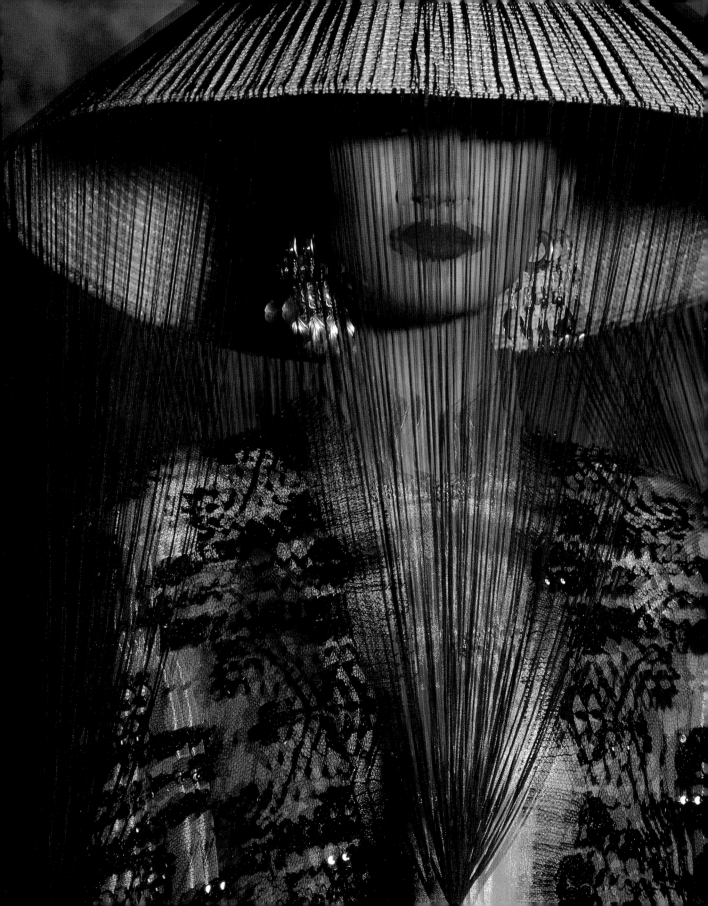

Inno Sotto

The Philippines

Inno Sotto's designs trace a journey through the diversity of a woman's identity. Every woman travels this path at some time in her life. His work distils the Filipina's inexhaustible source of romance. He skilfully combines complexity with serenity, while moving from young women preoccupied with the pattern and decoration of beading, through the lace veils of the mature woman's allure, to the aristocratic black-clad twilight of the dowager. Beyond the dreamy young girl is a stylish woman on a fashionable street, a corporate directress accustomed to exquisite interiors – a woman who throughout her life remains an imperturbable mix of princess and young mother.

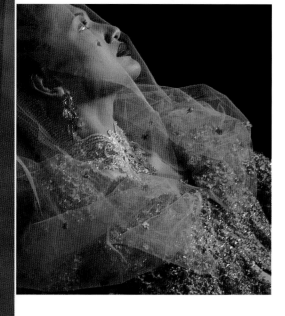

"When I was young I knew that I didn't want a nine-to-five job. My sister suggested that I take up illustration. At first I wanted to be an architect. Forms and shapes fascinated me, the logic of home design – why a foyer comes before the salon, or main room, and so on. I saw a connection between design and patterns of civilization. European houses reflect the history of European lifestyles and in the Philippines, the design of our buildings reflects our simple lifestyles.

There is a certain similarity between the logic of building architecture and the logic of clothing architecture. A good dress needs to be well designed on the inside as well as the outside.

When a client comes to me, I do not design on the spot. I have a little checklist of questions: Do you like a conservative neckline? How do you like the sleeves? How short or long do you wear your dresses? What colours do you prefer? This gives me an idea of what they appreciate.

Then I ask about their husbands. What does he do? Will this dress be worn for entertaining his business associates? Is he conservative? Does he want his wife to stand out on her own? Then I start to design.

But whereas a couture garment is designed like architecture, a collection is more like a performance. I like films, theatre and I love opera. The grandness of it. The richness. The exhilaration of the highs, the depths of the lows. Passion, emotions, extravagance!

When I was young, I was separated from my family. I tried to create what was absent in my life. My grandmother, who was raised with nuns and very Spanish in the Philippine way, filled our lives with rituals. There were fixed times for certain events – 8:30 for dinner and so on. The ritual of the table, no matter how simple the meal, was important to her, and thus became important to me. Even today I create rituals, celebrations of something. They make art out of daily events. **"**

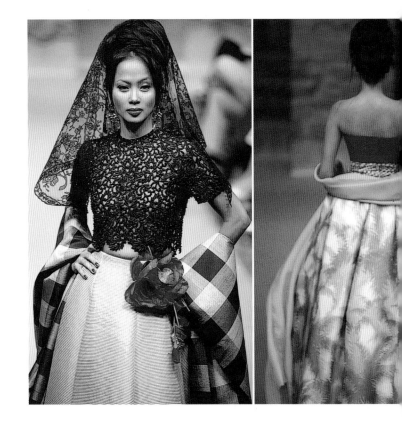

"Many things can inspire a collection –
a piece of fabric, a collar, a pattern,
an accessory, a shape I see on the street,
a painting, anything. All this is given
to me. I am creating for a purpose greater
than myself."

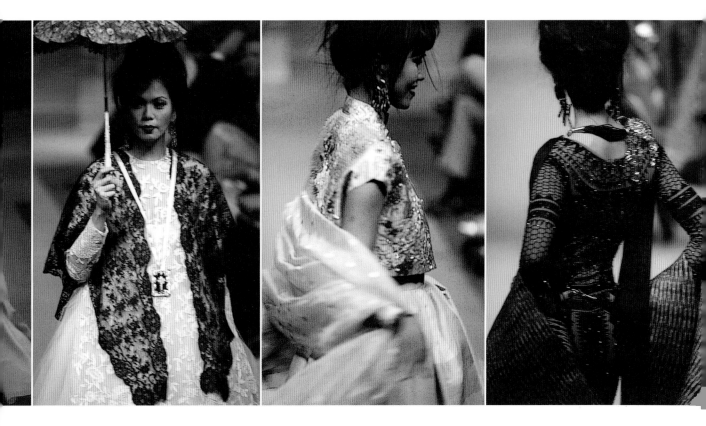

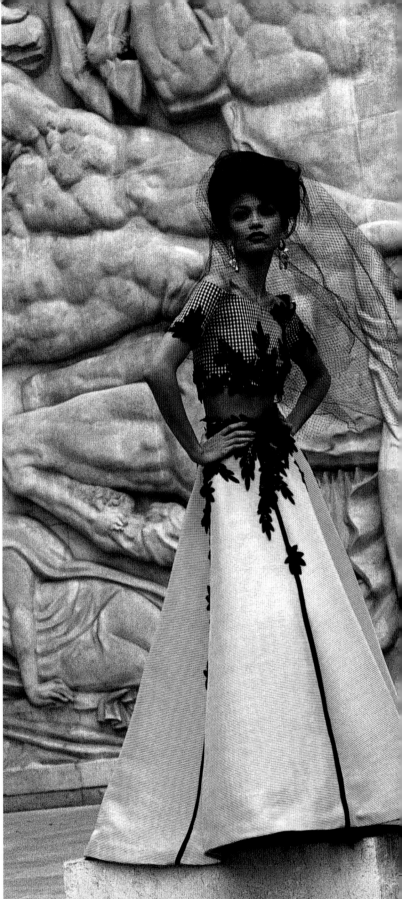

"When I design a couture piece, I art direct it: this is the woman, this is the occasion, these are her surroundings. I design accordingly."

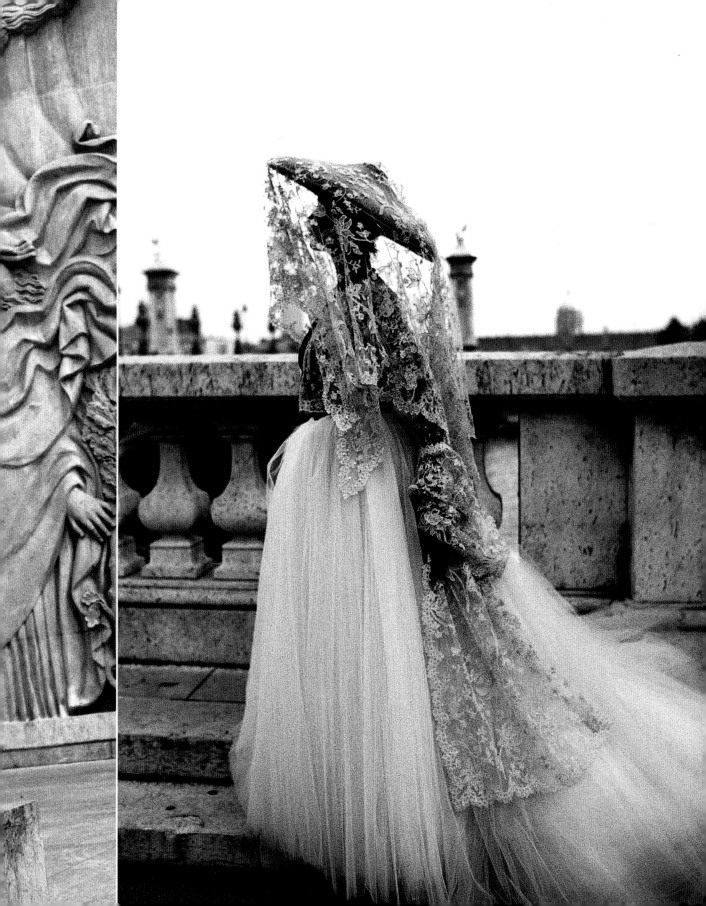

Patis Tesoro

Patis Tesoro searches for the unusual in the ordinary. She tries to integrate her discoveries into a sense of a new style using colour mixes, textures and patterns.

Her artistry hinges on how imaginatively she can apply her taste, skills, learning and experience to shape raw materials, or to reconfigure finished products, into a visual and wearable feast. To her, this is fantasizing with cloth. Fantasy not as frivolity, but fantasy as the outlet for individuality that customers seek in haute couture. They want a stamp of exclusivity which elevates their appearance into something not merely different, but so astonishingly different that it makes them stand out from all the rest.

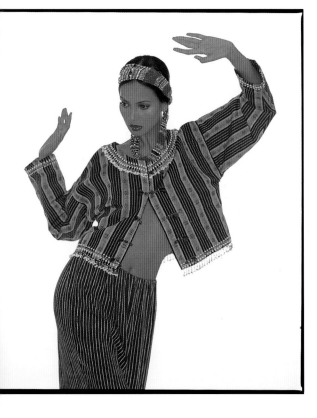

"I was born in Manila in 1950. At the age of three, I moved to Iloilo in the central Philippines (known as the Visayas) where I was first exposed to embroidery by the Assumption nuns. I married into a family that owned the Philippines' largest group of handicraft shops and began designing in 1972. I asked my mother-in-law if I could create a new line of embroidered blouses to complement the blue jeans that had become popular with the young. I started my own label, Patis, and staged my first fashion show in 1984. Since then, I have

"I aim for impact. My designs should produce an impact such that any observer will go beyond merely admiring the garment to inquiring about the designer."

"To me, technique is subservient to effect. I employ a fabrication method not for its own sake but to achieve the larger dimension that I am after."

presented collections in New York, Brussels, Osaka, Bangkok, Beijing, San Francisco and other cities. My interpretations of Filipino fashion were exhibited in 1994 at the Musée de l'Homme in Paris.

I was introduced to the world of couture by none other than Jean-Paul Gaultier who worked in the Philippines in the early 1970s with Pierre Cardin Manille, the designer's Manila boutique. Gaultier emphasized that haute couture absolutely must stand out and that a designer should strive above all to be noticed. Whether the response is positive or negative does not matter. What matters is that there is a response. Indifference is the worst outcome of all.

My interest in Philippine-made products is due in good part to my mother-in-law, whose passion for quality taught me the importance of dressmaking skills. My interest in indigenous crafts took off during my first visit to Kalibo, Aklan (a province in the Visayas) in 1987. There I learned that the traditional skill of weaving pineapple fibres was on the decline.

With the support of the government and private groups, I dedicated myself to reviving this unique craft. I subsequently organized the Katutubong Filipino Foundation, which is devoted to improving the lives of tribal and rural-based Filipinos by providing them with livelihood opportunities, while at the same time preserving their traditional arts and crafts.

Aside from fashion, I engage in product development and am deeply involved in reviving the production of natural dyes and their application to both traditional and modern apparel. In 1994, I published *The Art of Philippine Embellishment,* which documents my most notable designs. **"**

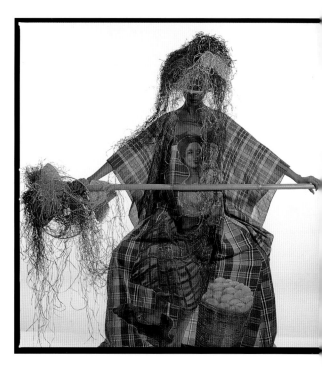

Taiwan

The Moon Has Power over Lovely Things

Design by Shiatzy Chen

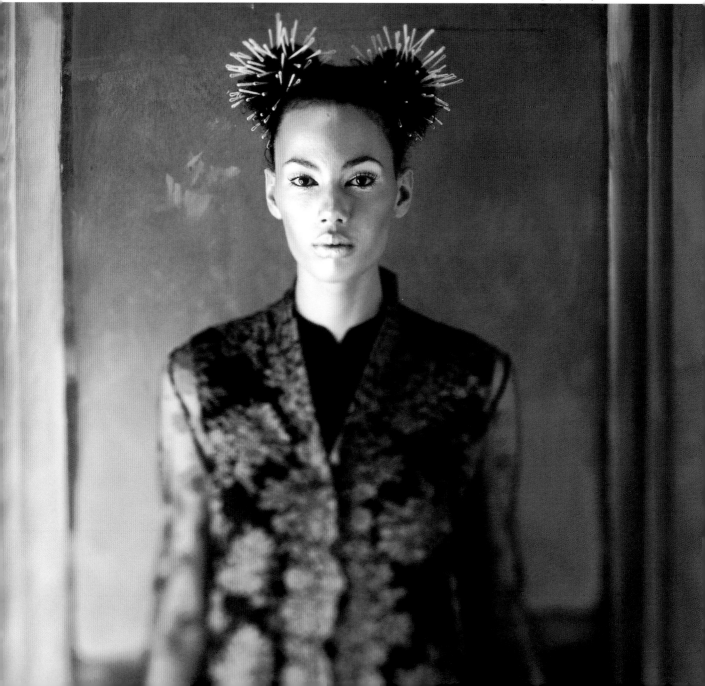

Taiwan is an island of the earth's most decorous hues: lotus root, purples, celadon, rice-paddy green, rose quartz. Except for the lapis-blue sea, there aren't many primaries. And except for the great tectonic muscles of its mountains, simple shapes abound. Light is adorned with leaves, sand, stone, sky. Beyond the crush of its urban cores, the island is a calligraphy of pathways written by people with their feet.

That crush and that calligraphy define the dissonances that its people worry about most. There's a feeling that Chinese culture is being lost to Westernization. People want to keep their traditions alive as best they can, but without returning to the encrusted garb of imperial times.

Unintended symbols of this can be wonderfully piquant. The one thing that the studios and salons of every Taiwanese designer in this book had in common was a large earthen pot with a single orchid in lush bloom.

I asked why. The answer was always, in one form or another, 'because orchids give so much beauty for so little fuss'.

Relinquishment of fuss to achieve simple beauty is a hallmark of the island's designers. The spirit of Taiwanese fashion can be described as backward-looking but forward-moving. Unlike the styles in some of the other Asian traditions – coherently related to folk design as in Indonesia, the profuse multicultural mergings of Malaysia, the grasp for the infrastructural future of Singapore – in Taiwan, garments are magnetic poles. Serene modern simplicity tugs back and forth with the thick fabrics and drapes of Ching dynasty garb.

There is such a lucid merging of the ancient and the new here. There are so many subtle quotations from the motifs of historical costumes, re-uttered in simplified modern form, that the impression upon strolling through a mall is that of seeing the ageing process in reverse. The adult arrives first, followed by the teenager and then the child. Complex fabrics revert to simple ones, colours begin with impasto sombres and end with the most delicate of pastels. Silhouettes recede from cloaky obscurity to the shape of a woman as curved as the garment can allow.

In the designers themselves, in the things they say about who they are inside, in the way they transform their feelings into objects that appeal to so many for so long, one sees the merging of mind and heart and soul and pocketbook into a kind of irreducible slenderness of spirit.

Then stroll the streets and see who wears these designs. Millennial ancestry, modern women.

The moon, the Taiwanese say, has power over lovely things.

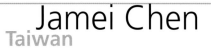

Jamei Chen
Taiwan

Jamei Chen's designs are remarkable for the many facets of character they reveal within a single shape. There is an ancient Taoist poetic ideal running through her work:

> Emptiness means nothing without fullness.
> Fullness means nothing without emptiness.
> They need each other.

To which she could easily add:

> One must provide just enough of both so each is the other.

The result reminds one of the compositional ideas of Toulouse-Lautrec. A large proportion of a design's total volume is reserved for the simplicity of things not happening. Into this restraint she throws non-primary colours and signature details, such as deep-hued monochromes and thin silver straps. Her details don't contrast with empty space as much as they add to it.

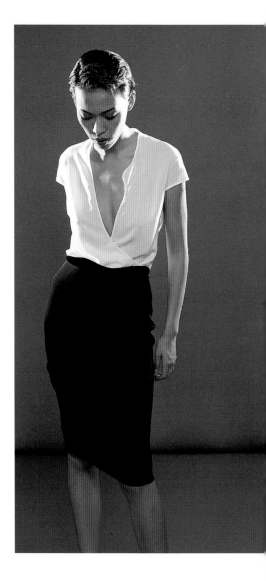

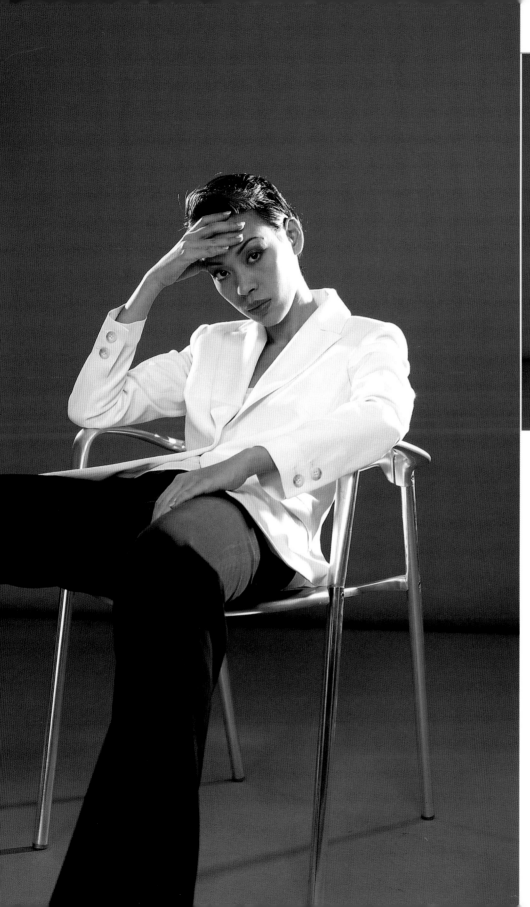

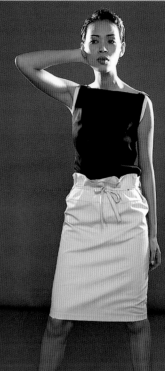

"My childhood was on a farm far from a city. I did not often see beautiful garments, but when I did, they attracted me like no other beauty.

My first garment was inspired because I could never find an evening gown that satisfied my taste. So my initial effort was an evening dress.

Starting my own design business was slow at first. In 1987 I established my Ji-Wang Apparel Company and created my own Jamei Chen brand. I wanted the brand to reflect my own personal style ideas in women's wear.

My line emphasizes simple, succinct shapes that embody simplicity as a high ideal in womanly beauty. Clothing is an art form with which I express myself. For me, the art is in cleanliness and balance. This is why I like the designs of Jil Sander. She is intelligent but not intellectual. I am very gratified to receive so many overseas orders from the better North American department stores. I am encouraged by the fact that I have struck a strong chord with women of serene tastes.

When I begin a design, I find the fabric first, then decide on how it should drape. My highest ideal is draping a garment simply and elegantly. Then I design the best shape for that drape.

I am increasingly confident about the future of the Taiwan apparel industry. Our insistence on high quality merchandise will be our surest guarantee of success.

The role of women in Taiwan today is becoming more challenging. Business has broadened our vision. We feel more and more inclined to wear a garment that expresses our own idea of what is appropriate for an occasion.

The increasing opportunity for women to travel has done this too. I am often inspired by the things I see when I travel. I can visit very different places, live in different styles of hotels, see different kinds of people on the street. All this can be more than merely liberating, it can be inspiring."

"When I create, I demand perfection and get it. That control gives me the courage to create effects such as combining the symmetrical with the informal, alongside the asymmetrical with the formal."

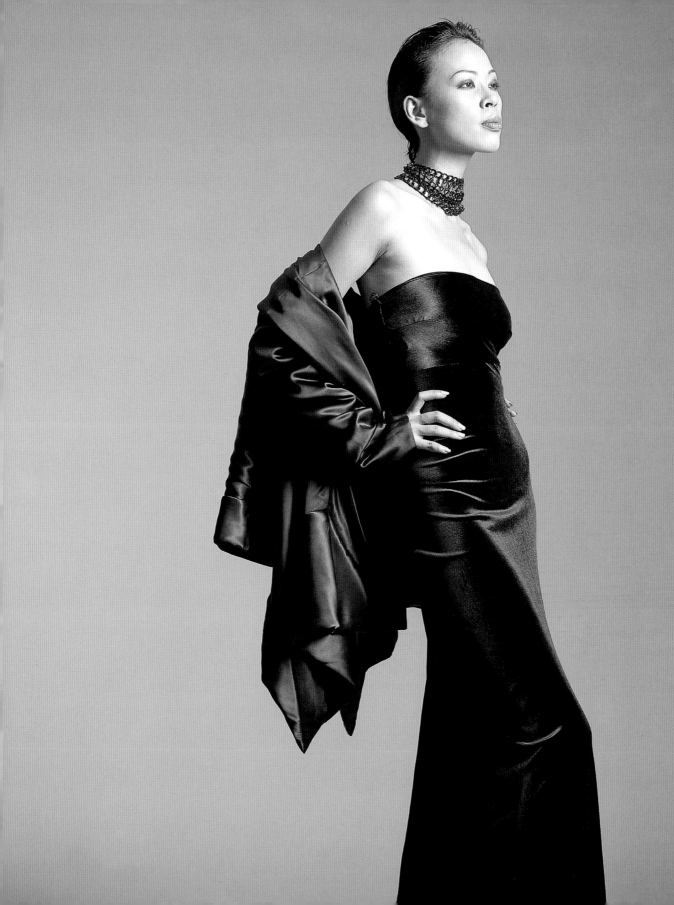

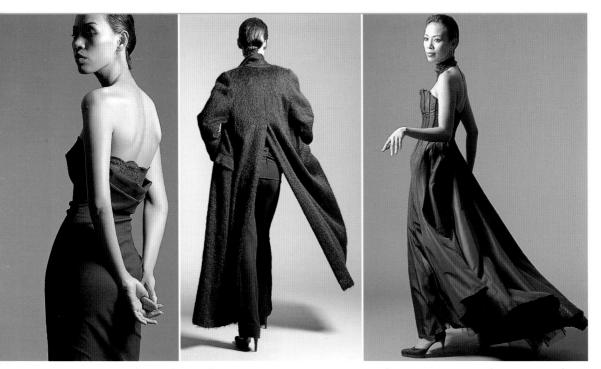

"The high percentage of practical yet also
beautiful dresses and suits in my repertoire is
meant to satisfy the many more lifestyles
available to women today. I intend to
continue designing beautiful, sexy clothes
for all women, not just for slim girls."

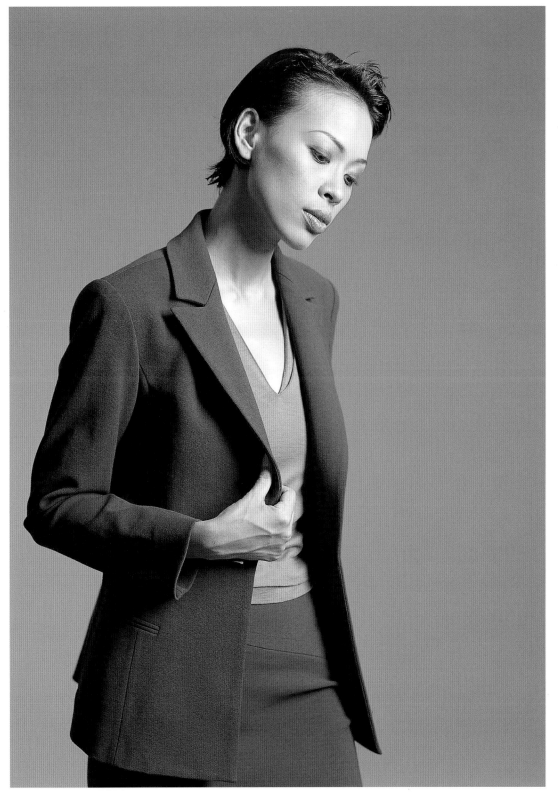

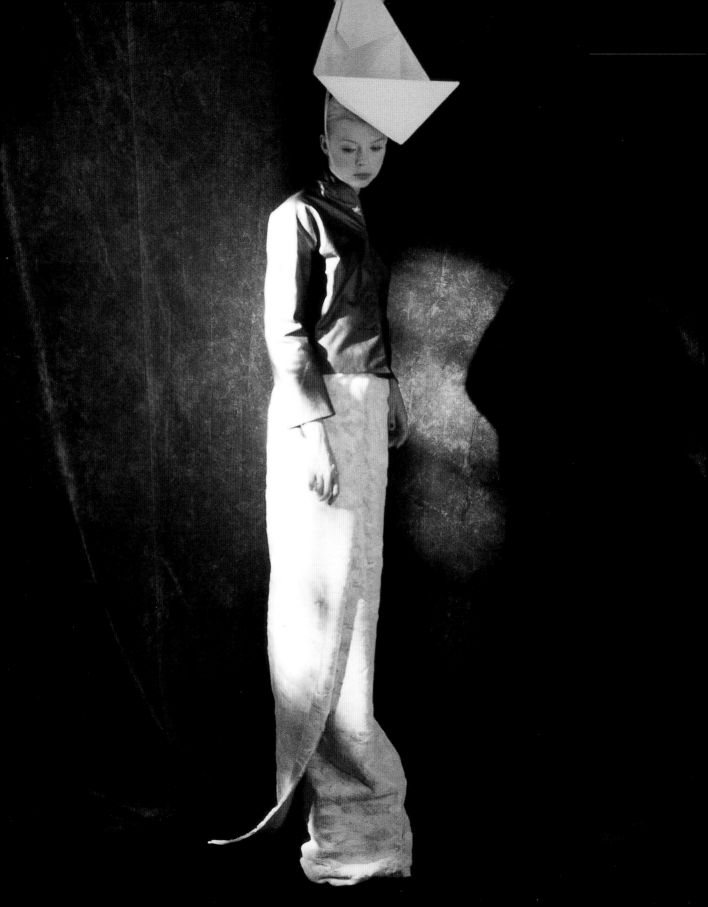

Shiatzy Chen

Taiwan

“My goal is that people will know when they see someone that she is wearing a Shiatzy. They will know from the fabrics, the way the colours are put together, from the spirit of the design.”

What happens to the artist who becomes successful at the business of art? Does creativity dwindle as the creator immerses into the minutiae of a company employing dozens of people marketing to dozens of retailers? How does she spread her artistic expressivity evenly over a collective enterprise?

Many people assume that the creative spirit gets stifled by success's embrace. Yet Shiatzy Chen demonstrates that this isn't necessarily so. She was an artist long before she turned her attentions to the world of buying, profit-making and selling. She is still an artist. To her, beauty is as much inside as it is outside. It has meanings beyond appearances. She knows that the problem with loving something is that too often you wind up with too much of it. She knows the power of the single orchid on the table of her meeting room.

“The most important thing about clothing design is the design itself. To me it is not important what dynasty or time of history a design comes from. The design has to stand on its own. Sometimes I put very ancient Chinese symbols – five thousand years old or more – into my designs. Only language specialists know the words the symbols represent, but everyone understands what the symbols mean to us.

"I want to create new clothing styles with a distinct, but not dominating, Chinese influence."

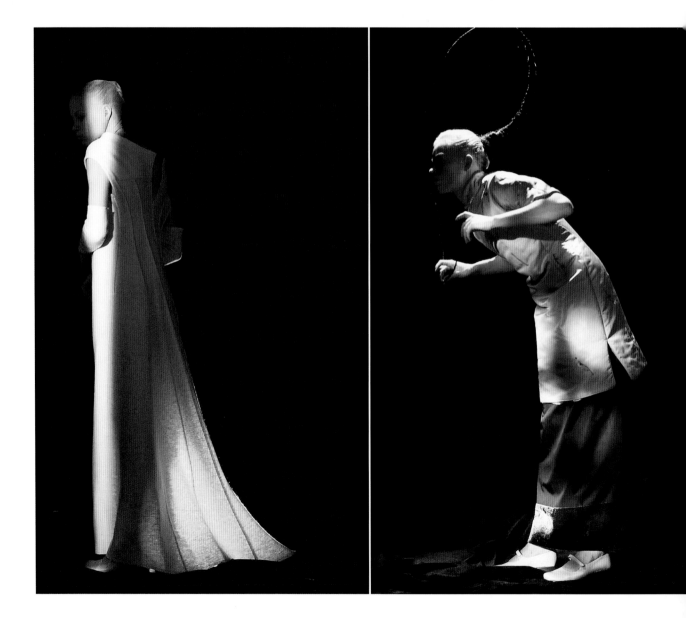

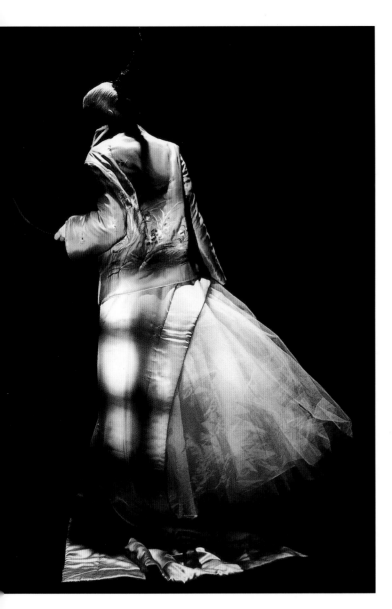

Even so, the past is just history, while modernity is history plus today plus tomorrow all at once. We Asian designers must develop our own ideas by remaining willing to change with the times. We must include Asian influences in our designs so they will be truly unique. We may try our best to combine the traditions of history with modern things, but there are big differences between them, which we must bridge carefully. I am still seeking the balance between market trends and my own sense of design.

In my shows, there is no cult of the catwalk or the model. Instead of making the catwalk jut rectangularly into the room, I present my collections more like dinner theatre. There is a stage with a curved ramp down to floor level and the models move among the audience. The collection is sometimes presented as a drama relating a particular story that gives a psychological significance to the garments. In one of my stories, a rich girl who is addicted to shopping learns that the joy of having many clothes is not the same as the joy of having many friends. **"**

"To me, it doesn't matter where, or by whom, the clothes are designed. The main thing is to make the wearer look more beautiful and have more self-confidence."

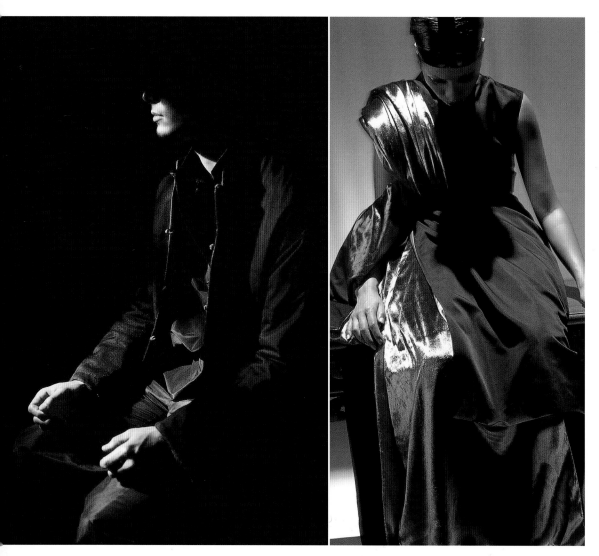

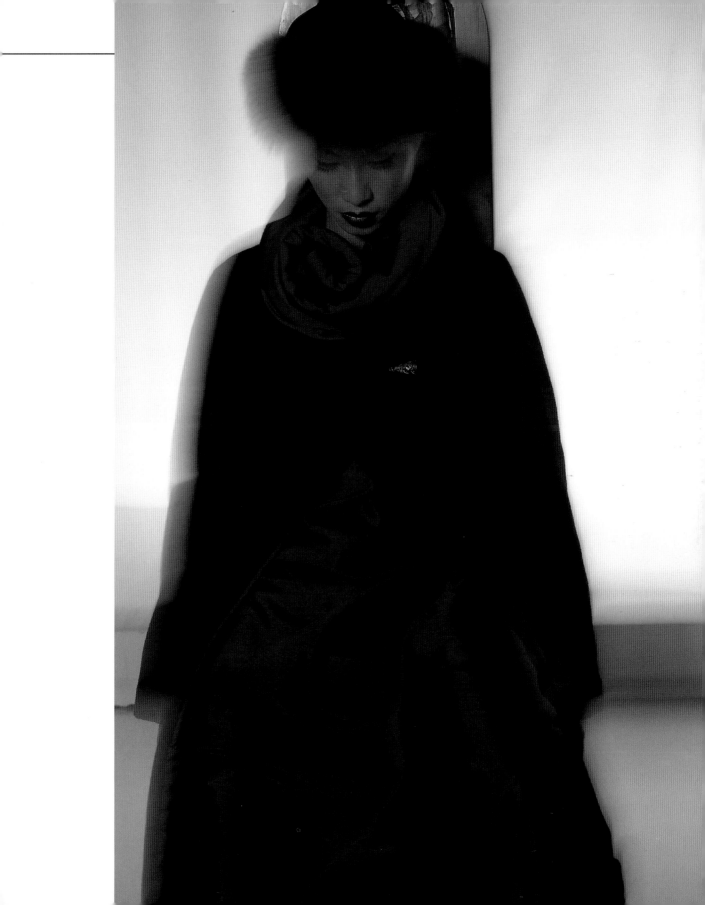

Stephane Dou and Changlee Yugin

Taiwan

Asia's fashion communities have more couples or colleagues working as a single design team than in other parts of the world. One reason is the strong sense of devotion to family that pervades the region. Another is the low levels of ego associated with self-expression. One does not find nearly so many titans as teams.

Stephane and Changlee fit very much into that mould. Both share the concept that the ideal garment gives people a completely liberating sense of fresh air. Most importantly, clothes should make people feel happy.

Where Stephane emphasizes texture and pattern, Changlee generally designs with more colour. She often uses floral patterns on the principle that if she feels cheerful with them, her customers will, too.

They are young – indeed, just beginning their careers. But already they are finding an enthusiastic market with people of their own age who want more casualness and spontaneity than their parents (and for that matter, than their older brothers and sisters).

Stephane: "In my childhood, I played with scissors and left-over pieces of cloth like they were toys. The shapes and the patterns of the cloth made me dream.

School gave me a fresh vision of what design could do to people's self-image and, because of that, I decided to go into fashion design.

To me, fabric expresses its true character when I use it in a subtle way. I prefer to work with cotton, linen and pure wool. The harmonious balance of colour, texture and pattern is the hero in my drama. To me, a garment is ideal when the person wearing it feels as if they're in a fresh new place, breathing a new atmosphere, when they feel completely free in it. Beyond fabric itself, I am inspired by photography and architecture, particularly modernism and the international style."

Changlee: "I learned silhouette from two-dimensional paper dolls, but the printed designs that came with the dolls did not satisfy me. I began to produce my own dolls' clothes by drawing and then cutting them. Later, my schooling taught me the basic concepts of clothing and the skills to work with fabric. It also helped bring out my creativity.

I'm constantly fascinated with the purity of a fabric. I like the solid but modest texture of cotton, the satiny but light quality of silk – for that matter, any fabric that can give a strong identity when sewn into clothes. Beyond clothing, I am inspired by animation and the movies."

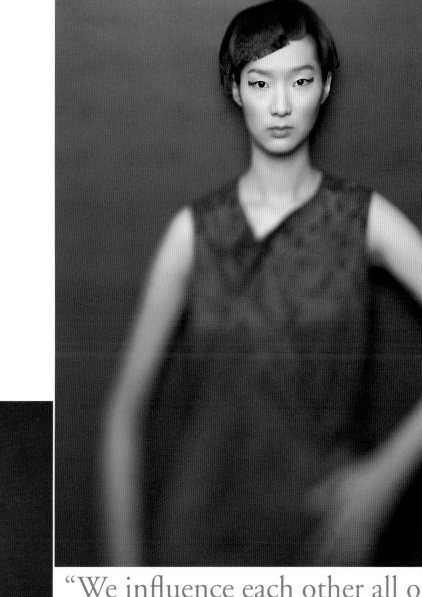

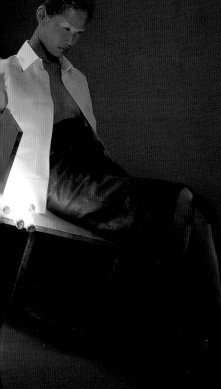

"We influence each other all of the time. Our individual inspirational spirit always comes when the other's is running out of energy."

Sophie Hong

> "Chinese silk-dyeing is very close to the ways of nature. If you try to dry silk after rinsing out the dye, the sun must not be too bright, yet it must be bright enough."

Sophie Hong sees women as bearers not just of children, but of cultures. She therefore dresses a woman for continuity, civilization, tough times and grand occasions. Her work is timeless and yet completely contemporary. Her work is more subtle than most people expect from a Chinese artist, her sense of texture and shape being more Japanese. She is after a modern international museum look, a simple, minimal, subdued but deeply textural character that isn't part of an assumed national heritage. She is not particularly obsessed with traditional colours or designs. Instead, she uses ancient silk-working technologies to create complex colours, which she then cuts into the simplest of forms. The result is not so much the shadow of forgotten ancestors as the remembrance of things to come.

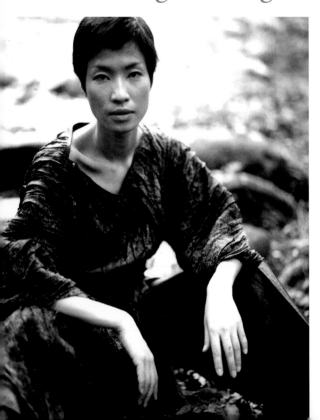

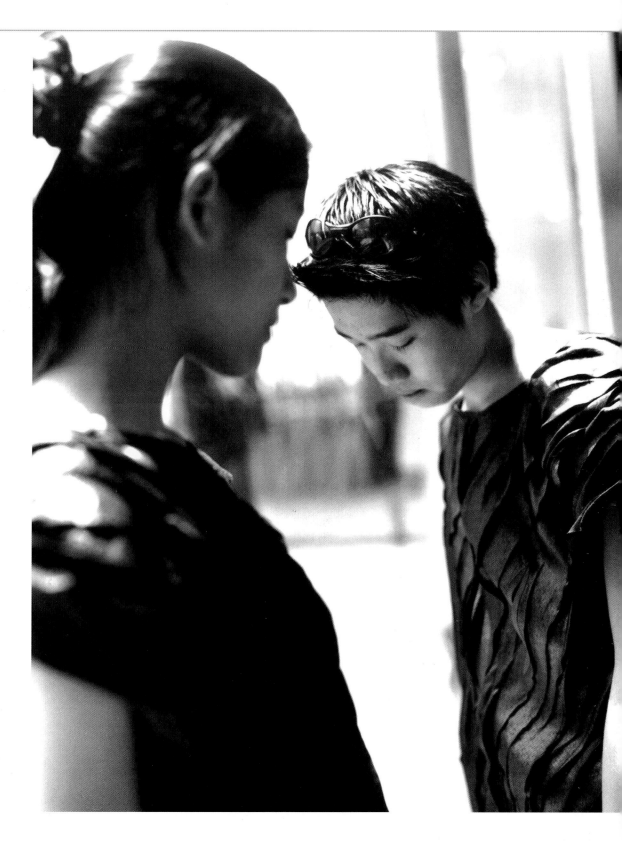

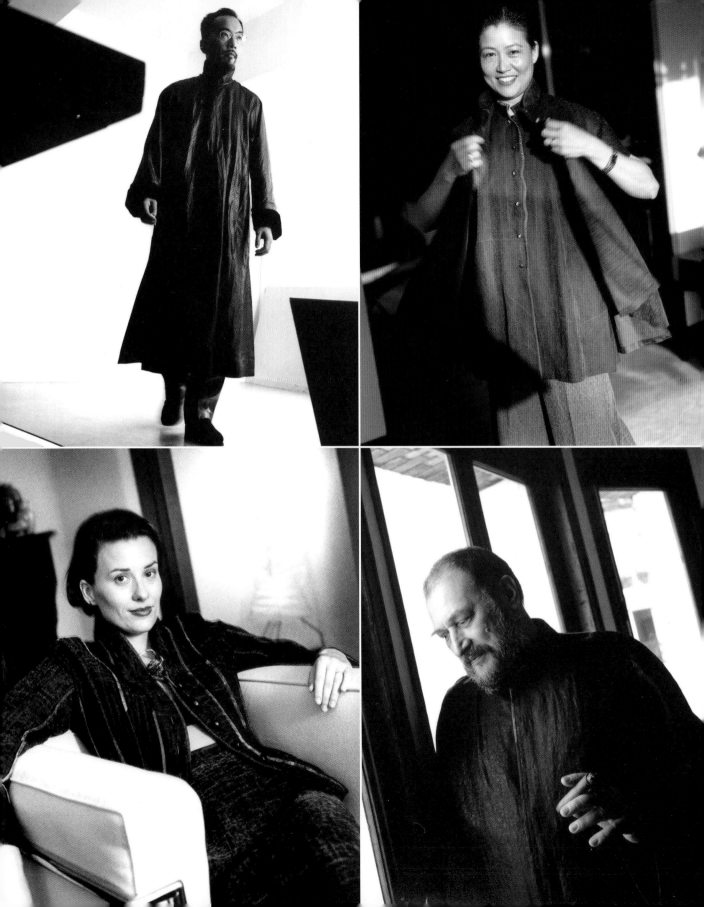

"There are good seasons and bad seasons for silk-dyeing, just as there are good years and bad years for wine."

"I was born on the seventh day of the seventh month of the lunar calendar, an important Chinese holiday. This is when the spirits come back to visit us. It was a festival of love and peace and goodwill, celebrated with firecrackers, street theatre and puppet shows. We had to make the spirits happy so they would not bother us the rest of the year.

From a very young age, I was curious about everything. Not far from our house, there was a community of aborigines. I was much taken with their tattoos. I spent many hours outdoors, in the water and in the fields. I had very few toys, but I loved fishing and watching animals. Everything I knew was related to nature, including the silkworm.

In high school I had an art teacher who taught us to look for the positive in things. He would assign us a subject and say: 'Draw this in five minutes. You must see the most important thing in it and draw that. If you

don't get it in five minutes, you won't get it in five hours or five days.'

I do the dyeing myself. The techniques that I employ have existed since the Ming dynasty. I use *Hsiang Hunan*, or Hunan Clouds silk; sometimes it is called tea silk, because it is washed in tea to preserve its blackness and brilliancy. Others call it Liang silk, from the name of the plant that makes it brown. It is then covered with special mud which, after drying in the sun, leaves the side that has been treated a deep shiny black.

Another method is known as lacquered, because you have to dye the material many times over. The first round produces a pale copper colour, so you dry it on the grass and then repeat the process. It gets a little darker each time, until, after maybe twenty or thirty repetitions, it becomes a very dark brown, almost black. Once this point has been reached, the material will not lose its colour even after many washings."

"I try to maintain the temperament of the East in my designs, even if I do not necessarily put into them the high degree of detail typical of the old Chinese traditions."

Lee Kuann-I
Taiwan

For all of the academic soliloquies about the serenity-cum-sentiment of the creative process, Lee Kuann-I claims that nothing happens to his mind at the instant of creation. He just creates. He looks at a fabric, works with it until it is beautiful, until he feels happy and satisfied with it. When he makes something, he very seldom goes back and changes it. The first time is always right.

"I was the youngest of three children. My mother was a seamstress. The first time I saw beautiful clothes I was filled with happiness. Even by the age of five, I liked to make clothes for dolls.

My mother didn't want me to go to design school. She wanted me to study electrical engineering. Eventually she relented and said I should do whatever was inside of me and whatever interested me.

I was first interested in window display design, not fashion. I learned from a Japanese teacher starting when I was eighteen years old. He gave me a good foundation in all the principles of design, which I could then apply to anything. My ideas come from the heart. Everything I've done with clothing design has been inspired by people and pictures, not from formal principles.

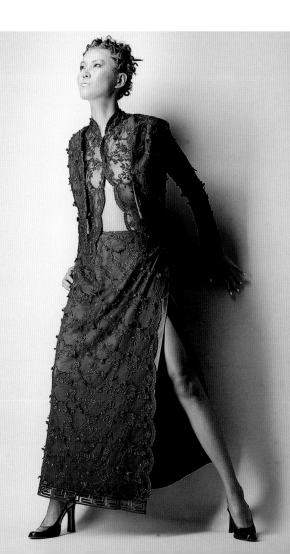

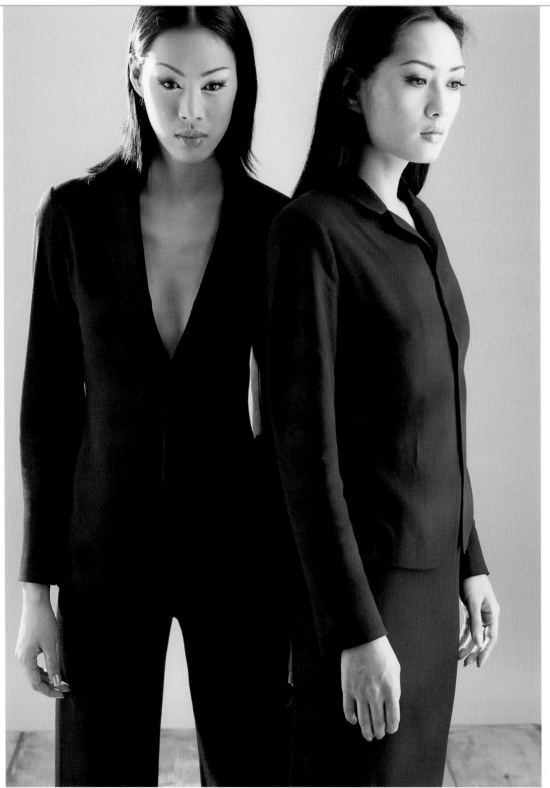

"I like clean style, subdued colours and cutting that is rounded and soft. Fabrics like silk and organza, silk/cotton blends, even wool. Soft, firm, warm, as close to natural as possible."

I met my partner at university. We had many of the same interests and experiences. Both of us loved beautiful clothes. After university, my partner helped me start my own fashion company. I showed my first collection in 1987. I did all the design and fabrication, while my partner took care of the business. In those days, hardly any men worked in clothing design, so I was something of a groundbreaker.

My early designs had a strong Chinese sense of meticulousness – rich detail, simulations of objects in the designs and so on. More recently, my interest in detailed surface decoration has diminished and I am becoming more attentive to serene line and shape.

My buyers' ages range roughly from eighteen to thirty. I design largely by instinct. I pay considerable attention to what is going on in society, the economy, government, the lives of people. There's no one single way to see the wearer. "

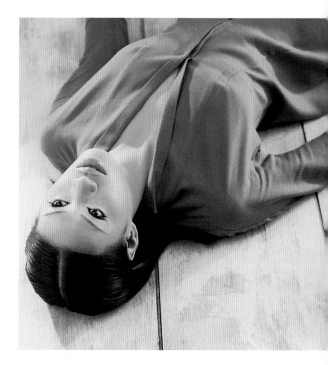

Hong Kong

No Place for the Timid

Design by Pacino Wan

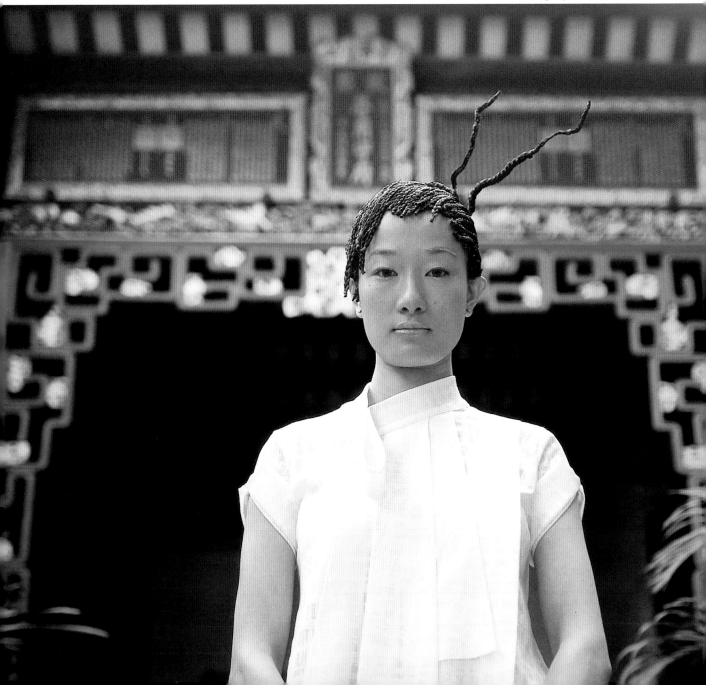

Hong Kong design has many facets but one constant: women are sculptresses of shape.

Here, taste migrates faster in silhouettes than in fabrics, which reflects the territory's established tailoring tradition coupled with its absence of textile mills. In regions like Indonesia and the Philippines, strong weaving traditions tend to evolve a less imaginative sculptural sensibility. This results in simple silhouettes, like the sarong and the baju kurung, but fabulous surfaces of pattern and colour. Regions like Hong Kong and Singapore, on the other hand, enjoy a strong dressmaking history. Their preoccupation is with cut and finish.

A less-visible influence in the tailoring tradition is that expertise was passed down from father to son. Over the years this led to a tradition of women having great liberty in saying what they wanted. It was left to the tailor to make the best of his resources.

Today, because tailoring is so often an urban craft, it is quick to reflect women's shifting ideas about body consciousness and, in turn, their subconscious preoccupation with fecundity in relation to economy. The garment's underlying principle is the circle of the life force itself: life implies continuity, continuity implies self, self implies style, style implies adornment, adornment implies attraction and attraction implies life.

As in so many places, in Hong Kong, shape carries not only the body's message but also what each generation foresees in its immediate future. The elder generation of Hong Kong women opts for a closet full of overwashed fussy florals, while the office-girl generation goes for sleek sexuality.

The Hong Kong design community's basic preoccupations are the relationships of structure to colour, of adornment to layer, and of simplicity to price. The 1997 transfer to China, coupled with the 1997–1998 economic downturn, saw all of these elements downsize. The shift in style appeared not in the length of hemlines but in fit and colour, ushering in a loose and subdued look, a kind of minimalism that allows a little fleshing out.

It is a curious fact that populaces whose ancestries are filled with vividly coloured cultural emblems are today opting for subdued expressivity in their contemporary wear. One sees this most clearly in Hong Kong and Singapore, the two Asian economies that are modernizing the most quickly. It is surprising how impervious Hong Kong young women can be to mother-driven appeals for timidity and how sensitive they remain to overseas role models.

Hong Kong has spawned its diverse array of make-to-order designers because its fashion customers are receptive to innovation. The rationale behind the success of so many galleria-style shopping centres is that the traditional department store takes fewer and fewer risks, while gallerias are filled with designers running their own boutiques in their own ways.

All these observations point to a fact that is true of Asia at large. It comprises many millions of people whose ancestry and geography organize them into many different niches. Hong Kong refuses to be categorized, which makes it a tough city to design for.

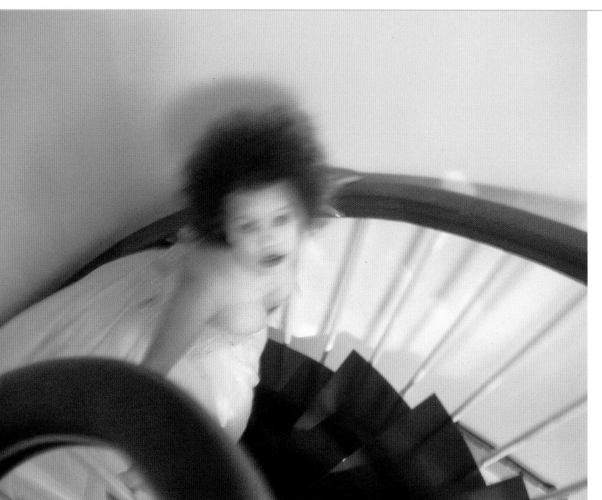

"My collections might be ethereally charming on one hand and harshly realistic on the other, extravagant or daring."

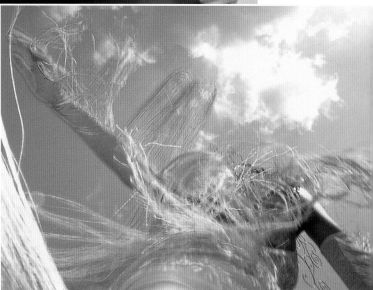

William Chan

William Chan can do the most improbable things and pull it off. Like mixing tangerine, mango and avocado with appliqué and wispy white cottons. He removes the black from a blackberry colour to leave an almost ineffable essence of pink and purple.

The results can be startlingly apt. Huge circular pockets on a light grey coat, with thickly woven grey skirt and sash over one shoulder, with the other open on one side like an involute lapel. A cable-knit skirt with panels of tattered wool snips. Spaces interspersed with geometric panels like a monochrome crossword puzzle. Pre-tattered cuts that pre-empt the role of time. Button-down chaps on a lanky leg, cut from thick felt with pinking shears. Revenge on the crinoline and hoop skirt demons in the form of a halter-neck top pinned at the back with only a single button.

"I see fashion today as the combining of individual globalism and global individualism. Fashion isn't necessarily style and style isn't necessarily a price tag. It should introduce new ideas about our culture. Designers should ignite a new sense of what life is about. I want people to let go of their inhibitions, be creative, be bold, be funny, be themselves. The clothes for this type of person should be glamorous yet comfortable, unique but what the heart desires.

I watch what is happening on the street, in the clubs, the soft geometries and hard truths of life everywhere. The psychology of everyday living and enjoying.

I turn my collections into the realities of movies, conversations, what's happening in Paris and the couture capitals, street rave, antique markets, the S&M scene, everything. I explore the metamorphosis of gullibility into purity, the twists and turns of tradition on its way to becoming modern. Conflict is a harmony waiting to be let out.

Once an idea is in motion, I go to the catalogues and fabric shops, choosing perhaps ten materials that excite me. I might change the fabric concept several times – a chiffon to silk, for example. Sometimes the weather can change my mood, say, from a silk to a velvet."

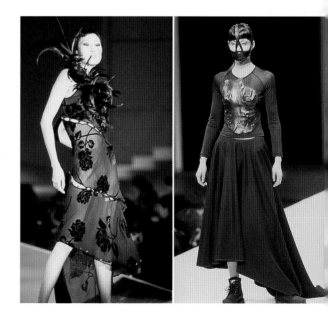

Bonita Cheung
Hong Kong

Bonita is one of the new, young designers who are making Hong Kong such an interesting place to watch. Like William Chan and Pacino Wan, her compatriots in age and outlook, she brings a sensibility honed more by contemporary media and overseas travel than by the tailoring tradition which shaped many of Hong Kong's more established designers. But unlike most the other designers in Asia, she concentrates on bridal and couture wear. Her clients have high expectations in taste and refinement and are among the most demanding in Asian fashion. Her success at so young an age in these circles bodes well for her future.

One day Asian designers will be regarded highly enough internationally to have monographs published about their work. Bonita is preparing for that by documenting her career with publication-quality transparencies.

"My mother used to make most of my clothes when I was a child, very often using the same fabric as her own pieces. That inspired my decision to take fashion and art courses during my secondary school years. Although I did not major in fashion at university, I always wanted to flex my creative muscles with clothing design and someday be in the fashion business.

A design begins when I first see an interesting piece of fabric. The touch, feel and texture lay the groundwork. Then I look at how it drapes and flows, sets the silhouette. The agreement between the pattern or print and the tone and hue of colours inspires the design's direction. This can be subtle and elegant, daring and bold, or clean and crisp.

I like to use a lot of rich muted colours like antique rose, antique gold, pewter, mushroom, mauve and olive.

If the wearer understands the work, she will know how to carry the design and enhance her own style with it. I enjoy seeing how women mix my work with other designs, how they accessorize the whole look. Usually the designer creates the piece and the wearer adds the style. Street fashion is often interesting because it shows how similar designs can look so drastically different when adapted by people with their own sense of style.

My inspirations often come in the middle of the night. I will jump out of bed at three in the morning to sketch them down on scraps of paper. Latin jazz that is passionate and lively but, at the same time, softly romantic is one of my main inspirations."

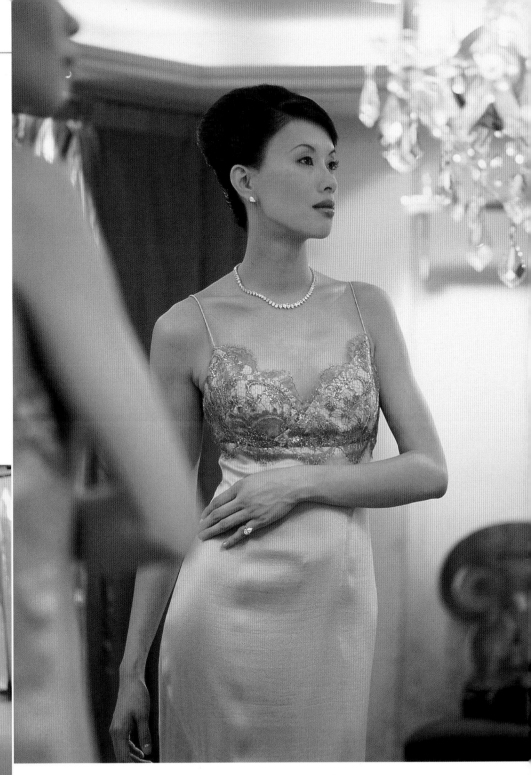

"I want to make the world a more interesting place with beauty."

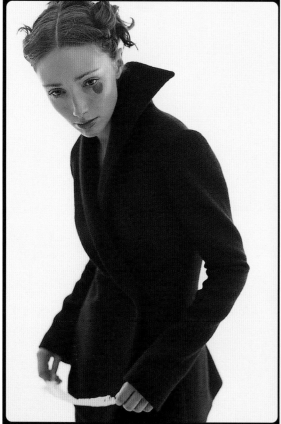

"I first let my
customers teach me;
then I help them
learn from me."

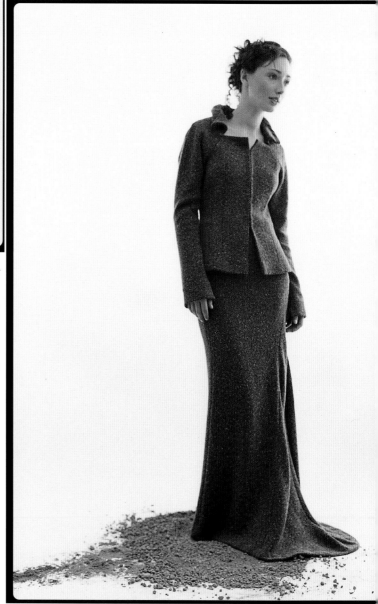

Lu Lu Cheung
Hong Kong

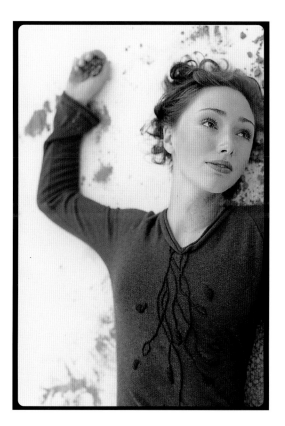

Lu Lu Cheung has a sense for seeing the significant in the swarms of images whirling into and out of the day. Her instinct is to respond immediately to the right significance. The result is a collection that is as much about Hong Kong life as it is a collection. She produces designs that can teeter between the cutting edge of fashion and the placating banalities of home – and make money at it.

She has superb diversionary tactics for making the best out of the midst of doubting times. Her clothes are like an affair that isn't about sex, it's about seeing and giving what the lover needs most.

"I was born in Indonesia during the 1960s. I came to Hong Kong with only three dollars. I started from there even though some of my relatives in Indonesia were rich. Chinese people believe you should start your own business and learn it on your own, not with somebody's help.

When I wanted to start my own boutique, I went to other boutiques and asked how to do it. It was slow at first because I did not imitate them. My work became very popular in Japan. If I didn't know something, I would ask and the Japanese love that.

Fabric has its own character. When I identify with a fabric's character the garment comes out smiling, like the fabric is crying, 'Help! Help! Let me out!' Character is different from a design signature. A signature can change, but character does not. My character is to see everything as a new possibility, then help others see things the same way.

My signature is simple beauty, so fabric is important. Simple is best. Colours, textures and shapes from the world of nature are the inspiration behind my soft and feminine contemporary look. Even when I use new technological fabrics, I line them with cotton or wool. I try to match the garment's character with that of the wearer. **"**

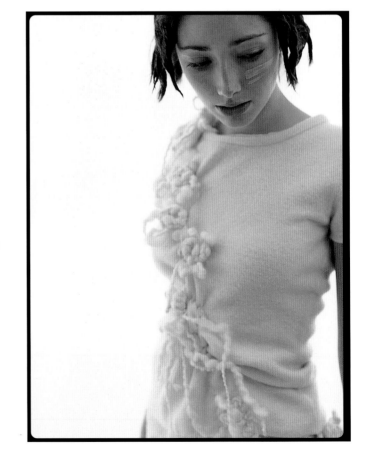

"Everything must have balance. The delicate and the strong work together. One must not be too artistic or too banal. A design must be interesting to the market, but also interesting to me."

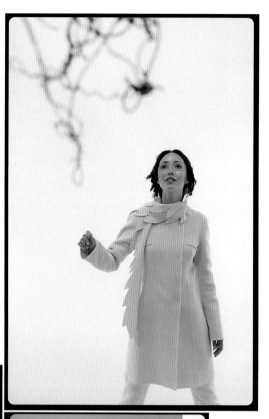

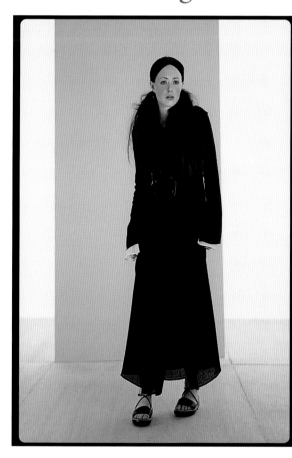

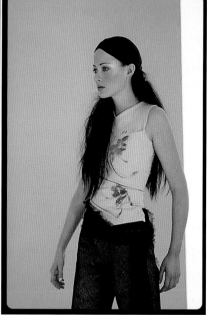

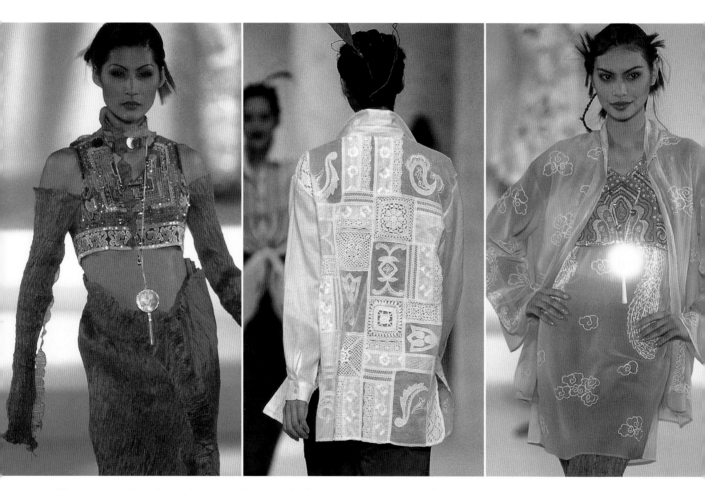

"Good clothes should contain elements
of creativity, wit, humour, know-how,
saleability and the pleasure of the designer
as she or he is working."

Ika

Like many of Indonesian ancestry, Ika goes by one name only. Isn't it interesting then, that so many of her garments are made of one hue? But, in that hue, her collection is theatre; it is costume as fashion.

Indonesia's history is filled with cultures of strong charisma: the Hindu aesthetic traditions that created Buddhist Borobudur; the local *wayang kulit* shadow drama; Islamic tracery in the wood carvings of the Malay sultans; the Portuguese waistcoat that inspired the baju kebaya; and the Dutch, the British and now the tourists.

Indonesia is not a country as much as it is thousands of islands, hundreds of languages and an unguessable number of cultural niches, little affected by the outside. Yet it is also a country whose people are conditioned by the constants of *kampung dan laut* – the village and the sea. The two are harsh worlds. The forces that bring happiness or misery are many. They do not emanate from grand celestial dominions with hierarchies of beings, but, instead, are found in local spirits, demonic and good. Each locale must live according to the terms of its deities. But it is also possible to influence or even control them by capturing them in physical forms such as weavings and masks, with which they can be managed. Garments, especially woven ones, become emblems of the weaver's power over the deities.

This is the world in which Ika moves as she designs her complex surfaces. If one knows the forces of nature that she senses, one can interpret her messages. The cascading waterfall effects of a multitude of different splashes down the surface of a garment evoke the ancient sprinkle charm, which reassured the prosperity of the planting season. The multitude of geometries in many of her garments – lace on crochet, pulled stitches, patchwork, lace, embroidery – reflect the tangled complexities of life, in which there is also great beauty.

"I am originally from Indonesia. The garment tradition there is one of highly refined weaving, embroidering and dyeing craftsmanship. This is expressed in intricate patterns and motifs, which I emulate in detailed handwork using beads, sequins, pearls, embroideries and a wide range of specialized stitchwork. A hallmark of my designs is the multilayered look in a single garment. I bridge art with what people dare to wear.

When I design I have a feeling of peace, happiness, excitement. I am inspired by Native American pottery, Greek motifs, Nordic graphics, the nations of the world.

I ignore conventions like borders and countries. Instead I think of people, colours, patterns, events. Ideas suddenly flow.

Good music compels me to create. New Age, jazz, ethnomodern, music from the south of Russia, good tunes from the 1950s and 1960s. What we cultivate in ourselves will never leave us. I love to talk about ideas. Just thinking of Kecak music and dance makes me want to do a Balinese collection.

Creativity is a kind of reincarnation. I'd love to wake up as a bird some morning. I love the beginning and middle part of clothing design, the creation and the

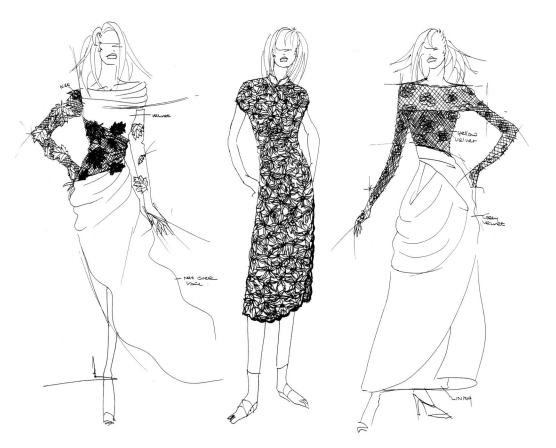

execution. The biggest excitement comes with the ideas, the dreams. By the time the piece gets to the production stage, I'm tired of it. Reality is less thrilling than dreaming. So although I never leave the art, I don't stay with the design.

I create from the walks of life, from nature, from the world around me. I'm an Aquarian sun, with Scorpio in ascendancy. Aquarians have a head but not a tail. They start projects swiftly, but forget about them just as quickly. Scorpios can be all tail and no head; they have a tough time starting but, once they get going, they can't stop. **"**

"My creative ideas come from colours and textures. Then I narrow these down to what is commercial. Sometimes it takes the factory and myself six months to figure out how to produce a complex look."

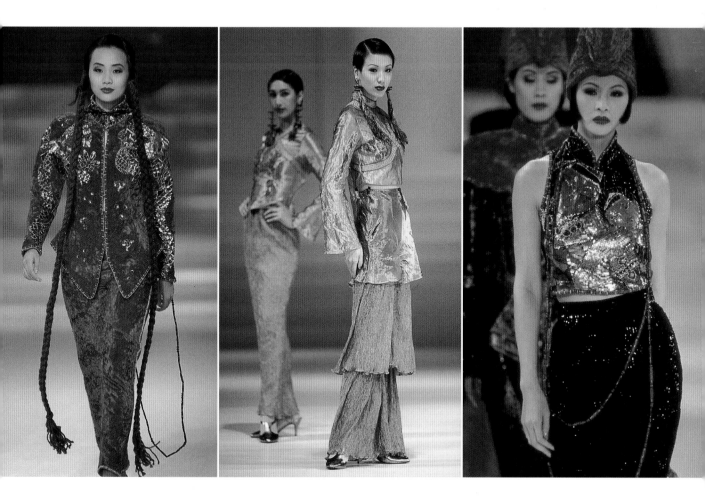

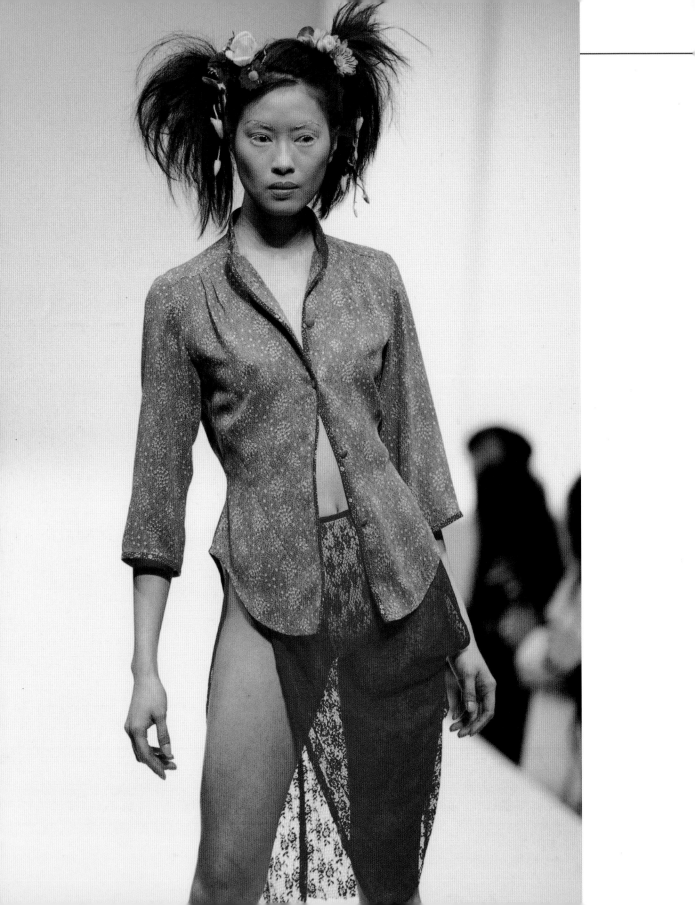

Peter Lau

Parents warn each other about clothes
made by designers like Peter Lau. They
do not like the clashing of his colours
any more than they like the noise their
children make playing video games.
Many parents think that classrooms
are not devoted to learning any more,
but are a computerized cacophony
of whistles, bleeps, creatures and
gadzooks. Youth wear from people
like Peter is scarily close to that.

His brazenness touches a responsive
nerve everywhere. Hong Kong's young
computer progeny are as preoccupied
with speed as their fathers are
preoccupied with predictability.
They are attuned to objects, megabytes,
virtual reality, morphing and Ultra 3-D.
Their parents, on the other hand,
are attuned to analysis, projection,
benchmarking and critical paths. Given
the comfy middle-class discretionary
affluence of these computer-cool
Generation-Xers, their thought patterns
are very different from what you
might expect. They don't think in space,
they think in time. Their aesthetic
impulses are triggered by events, not
things. They see themselves as the
primary market for the things they
devise – web pages, video games, jobs
in the new high-tech industry, and
their clothing.

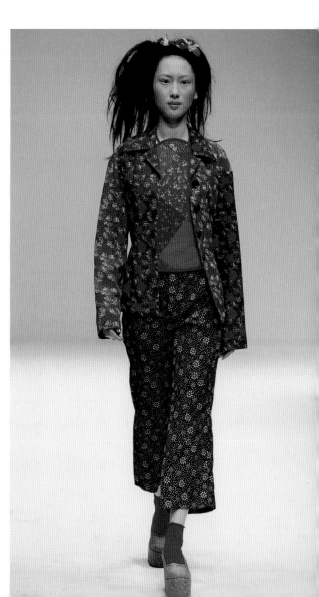

Serving such a demographic group could be a horrid style trap. Peter Lau's only lifebuoy on the taste seas of peer-group narcissism is his insistence on the continual self-examination of his creativity, of his ability to refresh buyers. Every season he tries to find new themes – a new fabric or colour combination, such as claudian red with orange, shocking pink with yellow, brighter than bright. Body awareness that doesn't believe in limits.

Models love his clothes. They never get to wear this kind of stuff in the mall shows. There they wear pallid mass-manufactured goods. But when they put on Peter's work, they transform into the sexy, exotic succubi everyone imagines them to be. No wonder the parents are upset!

"I never had any training in fashion design in the formal sense. I took a four-year course in textile technology, but had no personal sense of direction. Ten years later, I had a successful boutique and a very clear sense of where I was going.

I began my professional career with a company that produced mass-market clothes for America. The clothes used a lot of strong primary colours and patterns. My interest broadened into creating new textiles. By 1994, I had expanded my collection to include Chinese motifs and structures while retaining the feminine, sexy, exposed look. I added an urban-tribe look in the form of collage clothes – the blanket-stitch in over-the-shoulder cuts, the traditional cheongsam presented in modern ways.

I take risks with my philosophy of style which is devoted to neo-chinoiserie. At the same time I try hard to avoid the traps of style. I put my Chinese passions into my collections to suggest contemporary Chinese images yet with a global attitude.

I used to get my fabrics from European mills, buying at the Paris shows. Now I'm using more and more fabrics from China, such as the tiny patterned domestic prints favoured by elderly Chinese women. Their subtle colours and floral prints have a pleasant, safe, traditional feel, which is at the opposite end of my market, so I cut these fabrics into very daring and modern styles for the younger woman.

I'm in my mid-forties, but my mind is much younger. It doesn't make much difference how old the body is; as long as the mind is young, it will create young clothes. I will always be a designer working apart from the mainstream. I would rather stick to my own tradition than try to be rich."

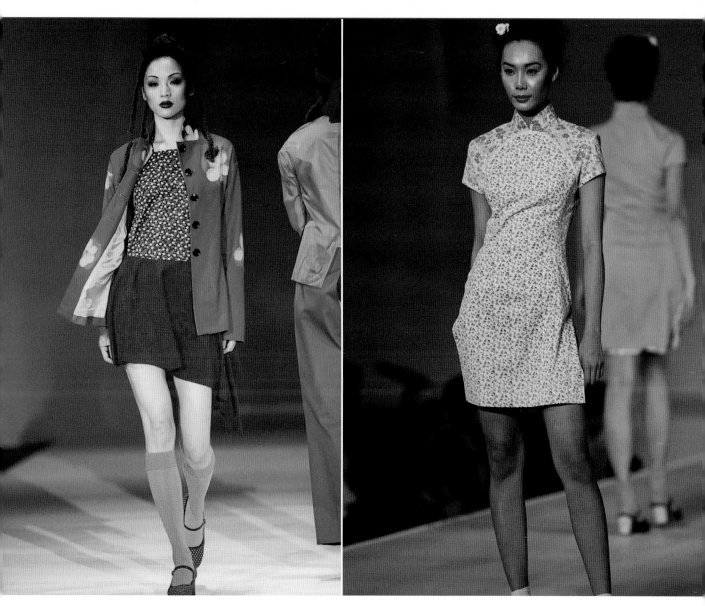

"The purely feminine quality in clothes attracts me more than any structural or formal elements that reflect clothing made for an occasion. I focus on body consciousness to accent a woman's best features."

Walter Ma
Hong Kong

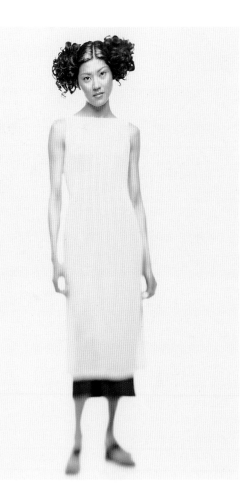

The New Look that Dior created for his 1947 collection was based on architecture and silhouette. Walter Ma depends on surface effect and silhouette. Patterns of blacks and whites combining structural complexity with unity. He can combine separates in such a way that each piece harmonizes with the others but translates back to simple lines and eye-catching colour combinations when worn on its own. He works almost completely with the mind's eye – juxtaposing, combining similar fabric weights at different scales, assembling colour saturations in harmonious ways, seeking common elements in dissimilar weaves. He goes for the stylish, fashionable look rather than the trendy, dateable look. His creativity is like watching a child fill with wonder as it conquers its fears.

"I started designing around the age of fourteen. I became interested in fashion design from the images I saw in the overseas magazines.

I learned about fabrics and dressmaking in evening classes at commercial schools. I started my own business in 1975 and one

"The best designs are the simple designs — simple, but not necessarily plain. Plain is difficult to sell in Hong Kong, but simple is always popular."

"Hong Kong women don't do impulse buying so much. They are used to buying things they can wear three to five years from now."

day I was invited to do a fashion show featuring designs by my dressmaking students on local television. Somebody called in and wanted me to be their designer. I was the first Hong Kong designer to start a label under my own name.
In those days imported garments were targetted at rich women. I aimed at the younger, lower-priced market. Not necessarily bright colours, but certainly sportier fabrics like twills and cotton on loose blouses and trousers. This was very different from the closely tailored clothes of the upmarket designs.

I had hardly any backing in the early days. I borrowed a little from my family and saved enough to do a small collection. I would design in the morning, open my retail shop during the afternoon, then go back to work again in the evening.

Media people never ask about what goes on in my heart. If they did, I'd tell them that the value of my clothes is in my heart. Not how well or cheaply a design can be made, but what the garment is in itself. I want a woman to be more beautiful and confident in my clothes than before.

I am inspired by no single thing in particular, but by the omnipresence of all things that can inspire. I absorb all the colours in the world around me at a glance. For me, a design starts with the fabrics. When I select them, I am searching for a new feel and look. After the initial inspiration, I think of the customer, then the fabric and the colours, then the silhouette, then the proportions. Today I have three lines, so I use three fabrics. I feel most successful when I see someone wearing something I designed several years ago."

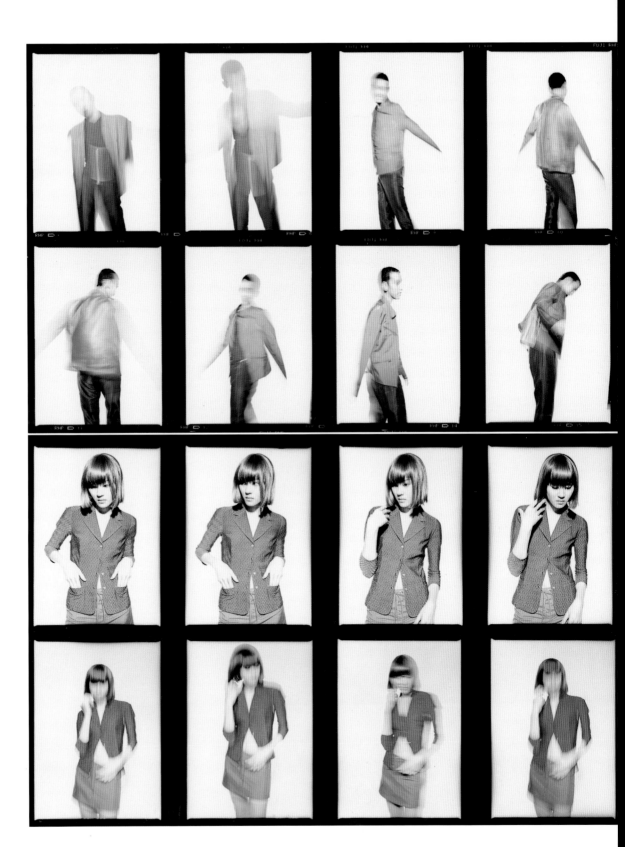

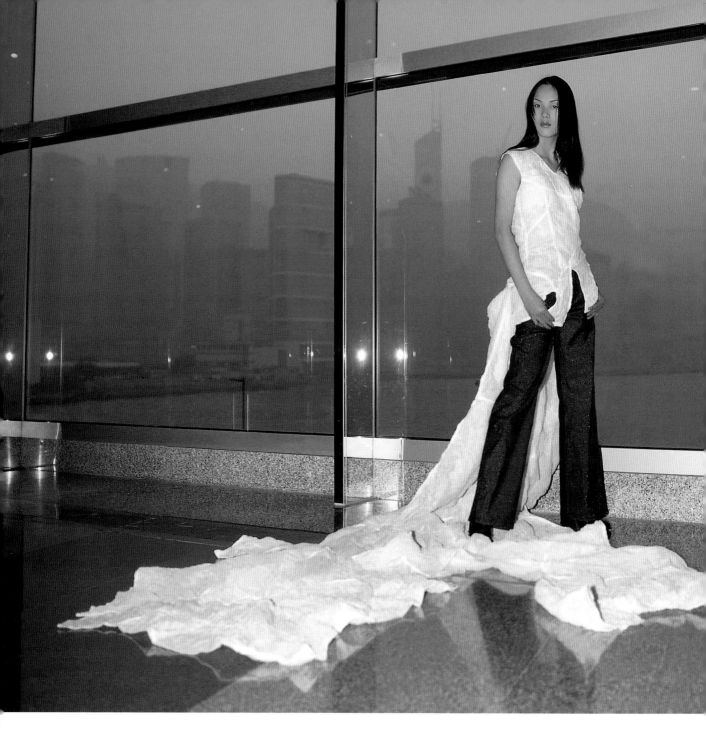

"A very large segment of our society is attuned to cut and fit more than to surface decoration and weave. You see more mixes of cut in Hong Kong than anywhere else in Asia."

William Tang

William Tang believes in the basic individuality of everyone, their desire to be who they are. At the beginning of his creative process lie two questions: 'What do people want that they aren't getting?' and 'What can I give them that other designers don't?'

He designs for people who neither seek an identity through the labels they wear, nor are driven by other forms of insecurity. Anything can be fashionable, but that doesn't necessarily make it fashion. One needs look no further than jeans or the sports shoe to see where trendiness ends and fashion begins. William Tang is happy with his life and tries to make clothes for others seeking the same happiness. The costume of life is like the costume of dance – it must endure tough times and yet come out looking good.

"I try to keep the ancient look and feel while not being retro. I conceal the symbols of old in the language of today. Many of my showpiece catwalk garments use long trains. These are references to the long kites used in Shandong province. At other times, I evoke the materials and textures of paper lanterns. This is an indirect reference to the light in which the kite and the lantern are symbolically linked to the qualities of silk and cotton. Most people don't see the Chinese heritage behind those things, they see a garment.

For me, ideas come from everywhere. Colours immediately make me think of a garment. Street beggars, graffiti, the changing landscape, train journeys. Early in my artistic formation I also got ideas from outside my native traditions. Once I saw some photos of garments by Mariano Fortuny. I saw his pleats as poetic, subtle, shimmering, enduring.

My family wanted me to go into economics or business, not fine arts. I knew a bit about garment basics from my love of drawing. If I drew faces, they would have to be shown on bodies and they in turn would have to wear clothes.

When I finally became intrigued enough by fashion to make it my career, I didn't have the mindset of people who graduate from a fashion school. I went my own way, doing fashion shows at clubs, shows for (and with) dancers and theatre people. My fashion thinking came from my association from a different community. I don't think much about social expectations or how people evaluate me or look at me."

Rowena U
Hong Kong

Rowena U's designs are sculpturally feminine but not too self-assertive. Her signature is the shape designed for fluidity but cut for comfort. She often does unusual things, such as asymmetrically cut, loosely woven (indeed almost crochet-like) evening gowns, creating an airy outer garment through which one sees the inner one. She has an uncanny ability to bring out the best contours of the wearer while concealing the not-so-good. It is easy to see how she is inspired by architectural form – by temples, shrines, inns and modern buildings – in her search for balance between height and width, surface and shape, linear and layer.

"I took night courses in tailoring and manufacturing and then a fashion design course when I was fifteen. I won an award in the Open Fashion Design Contest in Hong Kong for a simple, uncluttered design. That inspired me to go on to a fashion career, but my parents tried to discourage me, saying I would never make ends meet. In those days there were few fashion designers in the modern sense

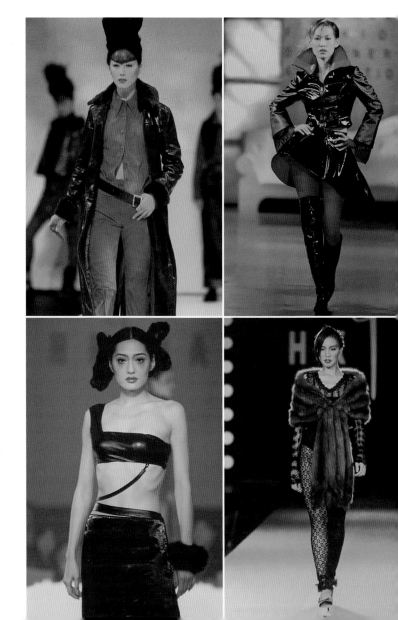

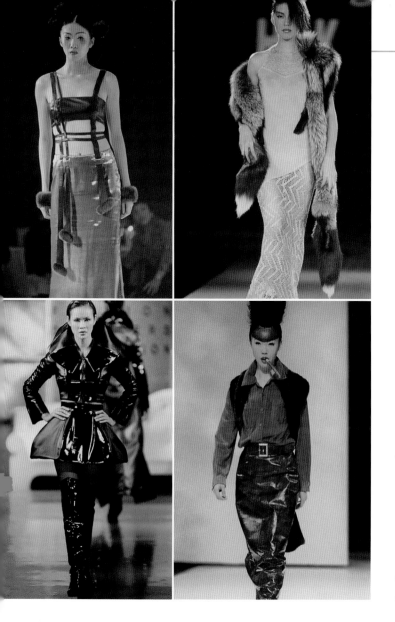

of the term. But eventually I established a reputation for the innovative use of natural materials, especially leather.

Over the years, by a combination of vision and trial and error, my husband and I have helped to define Hong Kong's fashion consciousness. At the time, the city was mainly a low-cost and rather uninspired manufacturing centre. Until quite recently, Hong Kong society women still bought most of their clothes abroad. Now they are wearing more local designers, which helps our international reputation.

If I wasn't a fashion designer, I would want to be a designer of another kind. I get many inspirations from my antique furniture collection, with its Ming chairs and old chests. I look at these and think of silhouettes, shapes of dresses on the body. The details of carvings becoming the details of a knit dress. Crystal, silver, vases – they all find their way into my design ideas. I emptied my bank account to buy one particular silver tea set.

Recently, I am most inspired when I am on our patio smoking a cigar. Yes, it's true! A good cigar is a philosophy all of its own! **”**

"What inspires me is the unity I find, the thing that threads together all the things that have soul in them. The garment is merely the vehicle. If I achieve beauty I will be with my garment long after I have gone."

Pacino Wan

Design for Pacino Wan is a balance between creation and reality. The garment as art does not usually get as far as the street (at least in Hong Kong) and he wants to see art on the street. In Chinese culture, a great many motifs symbolize luck. When Pacino studies images for his designs, he seeks out the age-old symbols of the gods and the emperors. He also uses traditional motifs, such as buttons positioned asymmetrically on a chemise, rather like the cheongsam, but in a very un-cheongsam fabric of crushed cotton. His shows are recitations of old myths in new forms. He doesn't want his fans getting fixated on the panoply of the catwalk, so he turns his shows into high drama. In one of them, he wanted to exorcise the idea of cool. He gave everybody a whistle when they entered, forcing them to be really *un*cool and create their own toytown music to accompany the show. The models weren't quite sure whether the whistles were for them or for what they wore.

"When I was young I loved drawing and painting but never thought about fashion design. My secondary school teacher told me I should study fashion at Hong Kong Polytechnic. It was a pretty breathtaking suggestion because, out of three thousand applicants, only 120 would be admitted to the foundation course and, from that, only twelve would be accepted into fashion design. Even before admission we developed the strong competitiveness we would need to survive in the business side of fashion design.

At first I was interested in traditional costume, but it was hard to translate tradition into fashion. Now that is changing. Some of my show designs are for press attention, but ninety per cent are for buyers. Almost all of these end up in retail stores. First comes the concept, then the details, then the colours for the season.

Most of my buyers are in the twenty-five to thirty age category and many of them want to look as though they have not changed much since they were twenty. The youngest buyers – in their early teens – still like the European labels; they need an

"I design to exorcise the ghosts in my dreams."

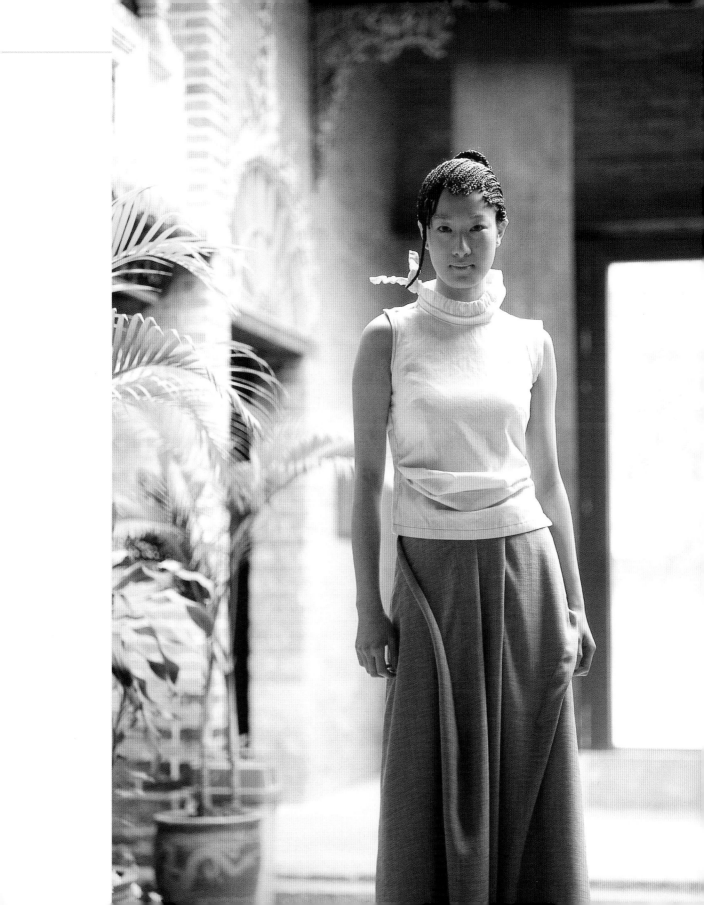

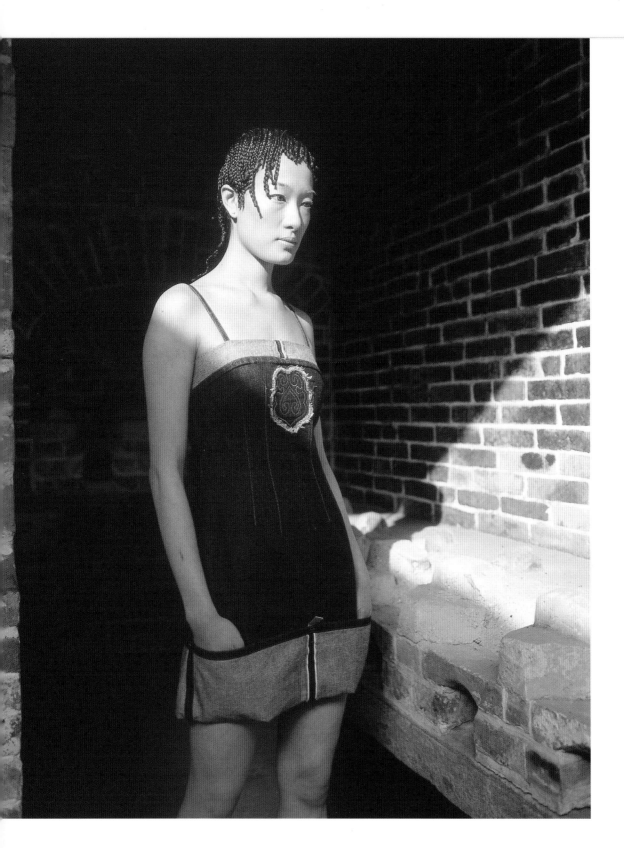

"A good piece of fabric fires my emotions. I want to find new ideas for it. Every idea is a piece of a puzzle."

identity and big names emblazoned on T-shirts are perfect for that. But when Hong Kong women pass thirty, they begin to go exclusively for brand, style and quality.

I design my own shop interiors. I didn't have enough space in my first shop for mannequins, so I cut and stitched together miniature copies of my collections and fitted them over Perrier bottles. The collections did away with the illusion of models, fancy hairdos and makeup, and focused on the designs and fabrics. My Happy Heart logo symbolizes my view that fashion should have some kind of fun in it. I try to put something positive in every collection.**"**

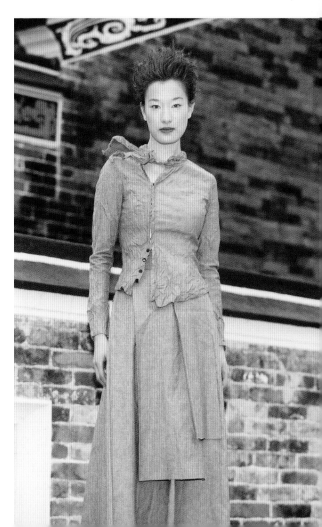

"In Hong Kong, people have little time. They don't like cottons because cottons are a lot of upkeep, ironing and so on."

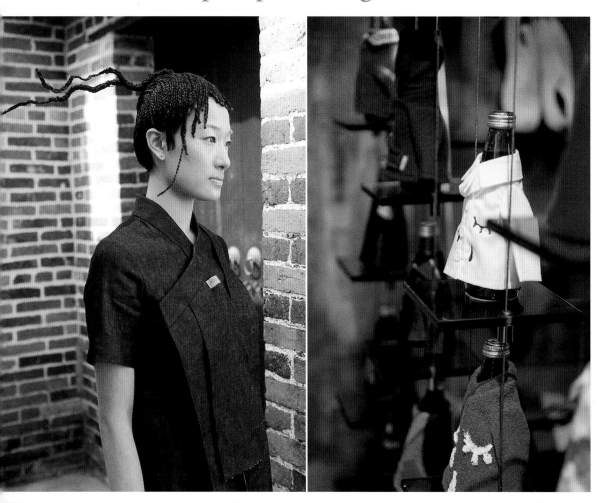

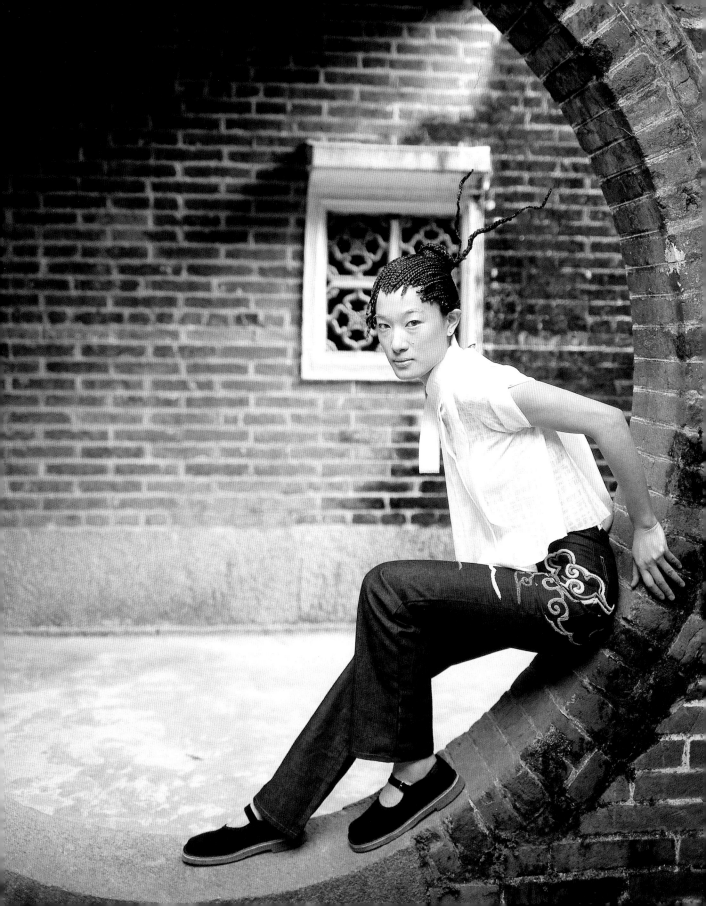

Benny Yeung
Hong Kong

No words can preface an artist, just as no historian, no educator, no philologist, no economist has yet articulated a philosophy of the garment, as it sweeps over centuries, or of the weaves and colours and silhouettes and knots which climb from every cranny of a woman's desire.

For Benny Yeung, a woman is at once formidable, fragile, fecund and fleet. Her beauty manifests itself in many different ways, like her life force waiting to emerge. Uniting this with her body by wrapping it in cloth becomes a soul-sharing experience for the wearer and the maker of the cloth.

Benny Yeung listens to her. Turning ritual into colour and shape requires a unique ear for structure, which has now become his hallmark. To him, colours have a life of their own. He explores the balance and imbalance they have with each other, the shocks of juxtapositions, the startling red dot that can totally change an entire garment, the delicate intimacies of pastels. His colours expose inner beliefs, communicate with the gods, portray deeper than decorative sensations – all more or less at the same time.

"From an early age I wanted to create beautiful clothes. My evenings after school were spent in the tailoring establishment of a family friend. The owner, intrigued by my ready grasp of various techniques, encouraged me to continue with formal training.

I studied in California and eventually ended up in London. I applied for a job with Nettie Vogue. The manager told me, 'Cut me a pattern. Right now. If you're any good, you're hired.' I did, and I was.

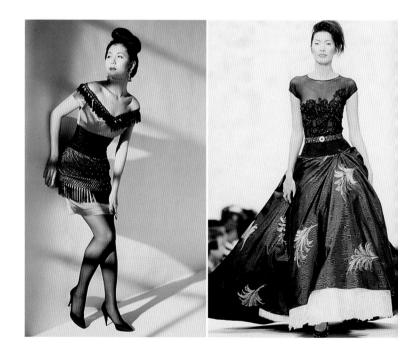

"I love drama and subtlety and try to mix them in such a way that they appeal to clients."

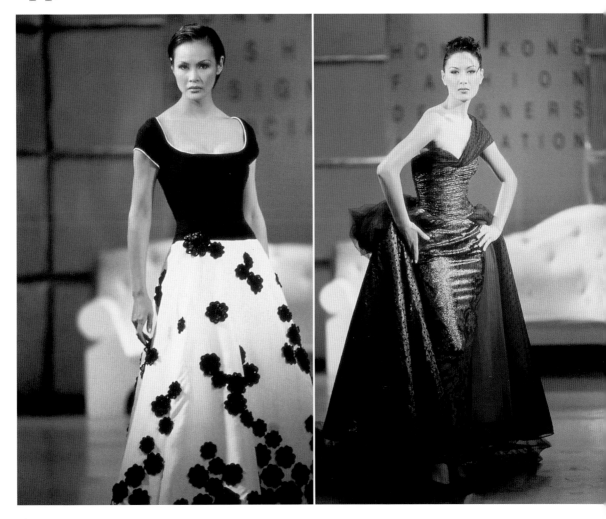

"I get my most creative impulses from travel, culture and old movies."

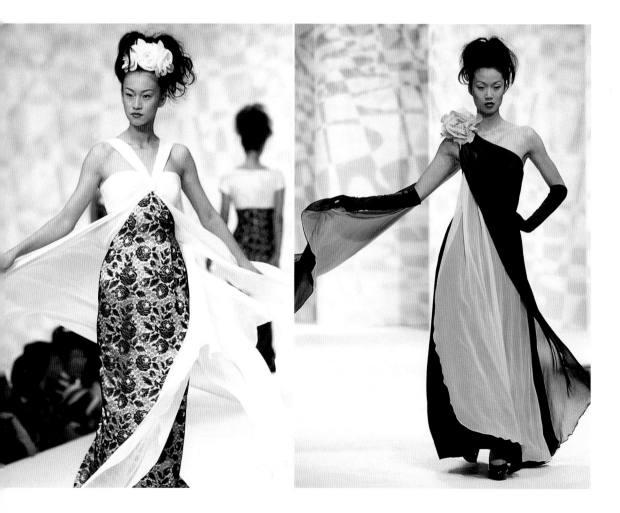

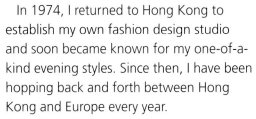

In 1974, I returned to Hong Kong to establish my own fashion design studio and soon became known for my one-of-a-kind evening styles. Since then, I have been hopping back and forth between Hong Kong and Europe every year.

Hong Kong clients like to see references to the past and the East-West mix in their designs. But I have to watch out. It's very easy to get too oriental – and even easier to get too Western.

I am frightened of what retailing giants are doing to fashion. I go into stores and see so many designs that are very similar to each other, and most of them very ordinary because ordinariness keeps manufacturing costs low. Too many customers get their ideas from magazines without developing their own sensibilities.

Fashion journalists sometimes criticize a collection without being able to identify the reasons why this or that garment was designed the way it was. An ignorant media writer can blunderingly trample a refined collection.

Older customers are now looking for clothes that stay fashionable for a long time. Younger buyers are interested in a more quickly moving style. Students are coming up with some good ideas, but don't get enough practical training. Many are good on sketches, but lack either a sophisticated knowledge of fabrics or a sense of the social needs of the client. "

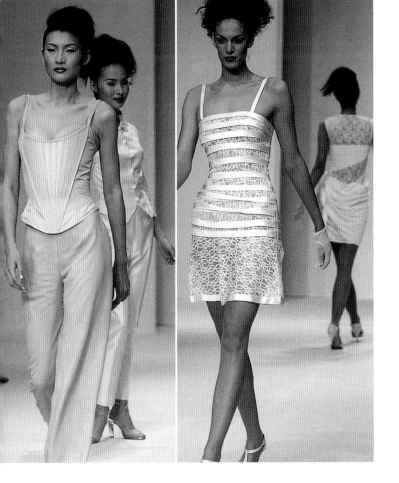

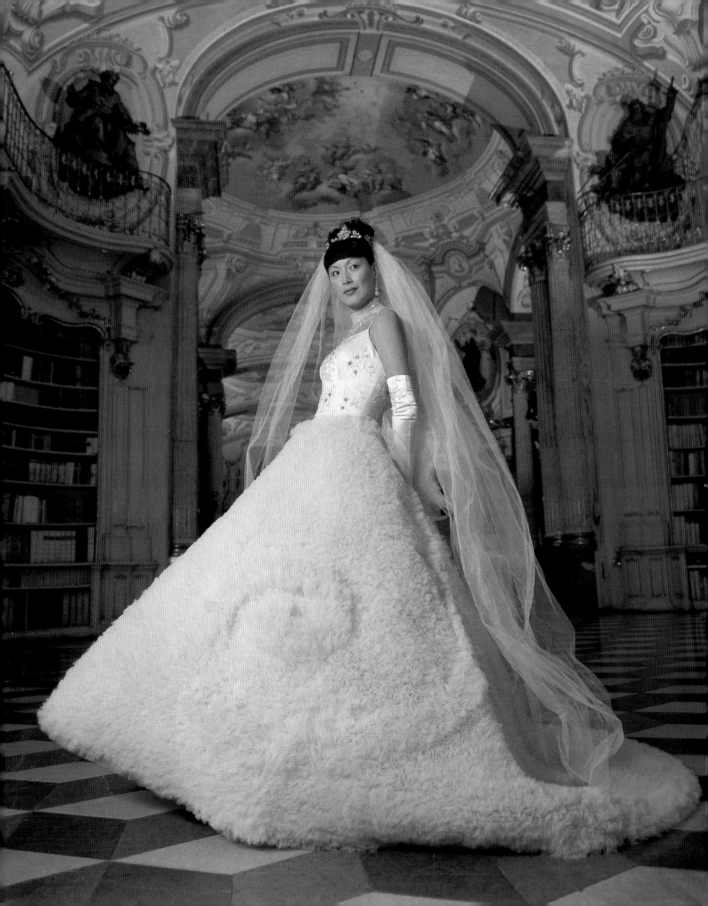

Kevin Yeung
Hong Kong

"The design is either correct at the first snip of the scissors, or it will never be right."

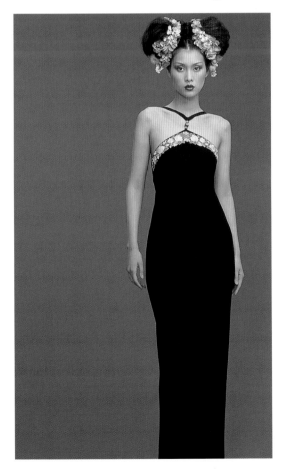

Kevin Yeung sees himself as the middle ground between the fabric and the garment. He starts with 'What if?', a vague concept of the garment he wants, and keeps asking 'Why not?' But when he flattens the cloth on the table in front of him, he cuts without hesitation.

He has always been close to the business side of the fashion world, as well as basking in the fame and fun of being a designer. His organizational skills are so much in demand that he has been chairman of the Hong Kong Fashion Designers Association since 1996.

"I first knew I wanted to be a fashion designer when I was a young boy. I liked drawing a lot, but didn't have any opportunity to train professionally. Thirty years ago there was no fashion school in Hong Kong. People thought that it was not a secure profession and therefore not prestigious. Today we have Hong Kong Polytechnic.

> "To me, fashion is a way of life. Clothes should make a statement about your lifestyle. They should not overwhelm your personality."

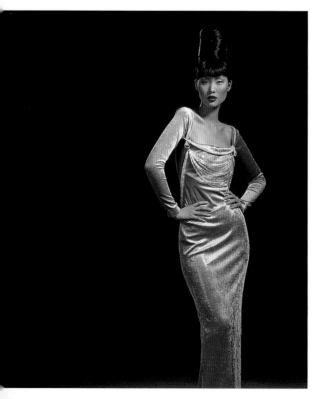

In 1974 I studied fashion design for two years in Paris. The French teaching style was to drape fabrics on a dummy to create the design. They didn't cut patterns until after the design was established and they needed to scale it up or down. This taught me to think on the body, not on paper.

I started a shop selling designs to commercial fashion houses in the mid-1970s. It was fairly lucrative for the amount of work involved. In those days, commercial manufacturers would buy designs from independents rather than employing in-house designers. The official price was 500 francs. But, all too often, I had to sell many of my designs for only 200 francs to make ends meet.

I returned to Hong Kong and started a boutique, which lasted for three years. Those years taught me that the boutique business is not that interesting – I had to be salesman, businessman, accountant and, only after all that, a designer. A Canadian company asked me to be their designer. It was unusual for an overseas firm to hire a Hong Kong designer, but the company thrived on my collections and, after two years, I was promoted to chief designer.

I quit to start my Gobelins company, naming it after the 13th arrondissement in Paris where I once lived. I started with executive wear but moved on to party dresses. These require a lot of time to get the perfect cut and style, but are quite satisfying to do. We went into evening gowns and now I have customers in Hong Kong, Japan and Paris. **"**

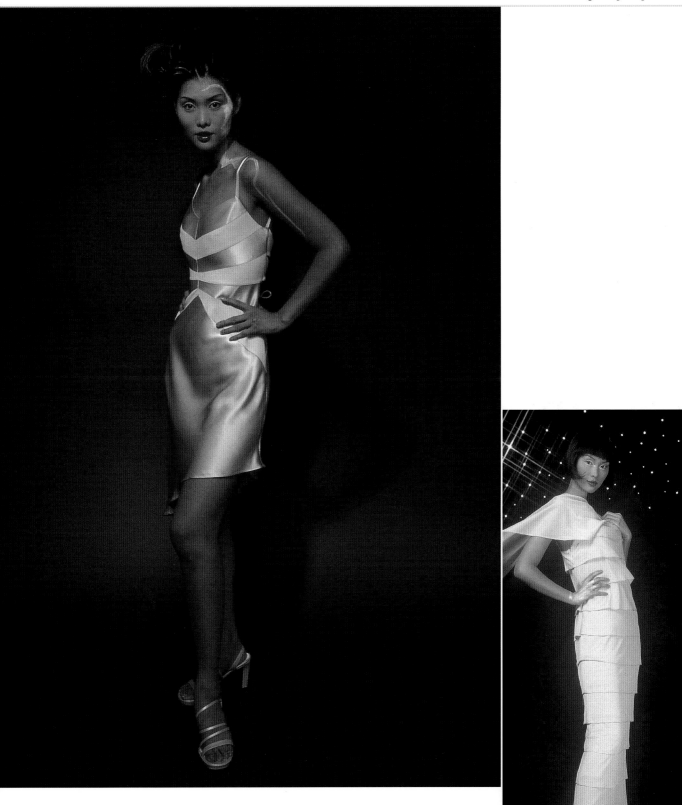

Riddle in a Mystery in an Enigma

Design by Coco Ma

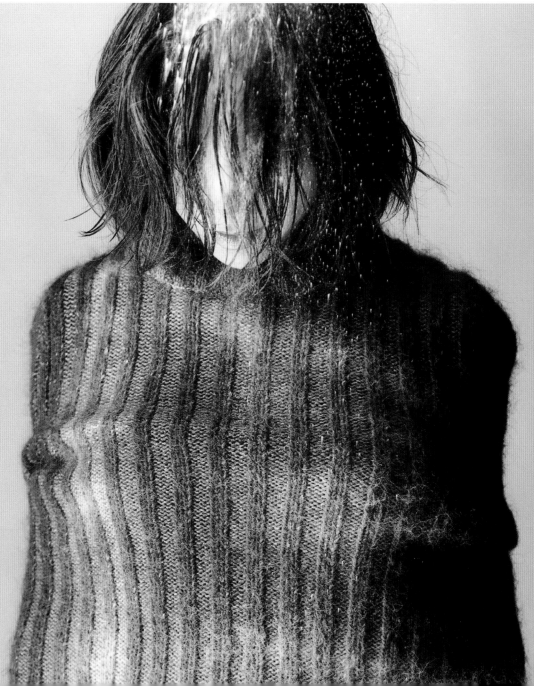

The future of Chinese fashion is the big question mark hovering over the future of Asian fashion design. At present, that question mark is economic. China's productivity power and labour costs are so low that the country's garment industry can easily overwhelm its regional compatriots in export sales to Europe and the Americas – and indeed, even within Asia itself. It is ominous to walk through the malls of Asia's cities and see how often the 'Made in China' label is stitched to the cheapest items. And unlike the Asia of old, low price is no longer a byword for shoddy quality.

But garments are not fashion. The Maoist attempt to channel urban creative ideation into rural grindstone labour surely extinguished all but a very few roots of the innovation tree. Worse, Maoism erased the market for such things.

The enigma in the title of this chapter therefore lies in the extent to which the roots survived. The best assessment so far would be to say widely, but not deeply. The single outstanding characteristic of the Chinese designers interviewed here was the sincerity of their modesty. When Coco Ma speaks of how she talked to a kitten in Hong Kong, the hip fashion world will grimace at the candour of such naivety. And yet she is more principled in her honesty than those who laugh.

Coco Ma is but one example. Yvoone Ding Xue Lian is another and for a very different reason. She represents the mystery in our title. The only work she could supply for consideration were her sketches. She could proffer few photographs. Why? Her employer is a state-owned corporation that could not visualize the boon to them of Yvoone Ding Xue Lian being in a book like this. So we never got any pictures.

One has to admire people like Yvoone Ding Xue Lian and Coco Ma. They face economic constraints that few designers in this book have endured. As yet, they have little freedom to do anything beyond what their perceived market demands. The mystery lies in how they have managed to do so well with so little, since their work certainly equals the everyday ware in Asia's malls.

And on to the riddle. When will this change? When will China's designers be able to express themselves as freely as, say, Hong Kong's? Assuredly, the market exists. The social events of Beijing and Shanghai are dotted with women who express their good taste in the way they dress. Some have their clothes tailored locally, thus keeping alive that most ancient of China's garbing traditions. Others buy foreign, no matter the cost (indeed, often because of it).

There are two faces to this riddle. On one side, the economic situation of the state-owned companies is so difficult that the designers cannot think of frills at a time like this. On the other, if they aren't creative and if they don't enter the mainstream of Asian fashion, their cost advantage will slip away.

So while there are designers who constitute living answers to the mystery and to the enigma, there are no solutions to the riddle. Instead, it prompts yet another question that applies to all of Asia. If economies don't last forever, how do you plan for the future? Will quantity be the saving grace, or will it be quality?

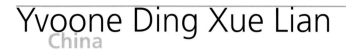

Yvoone Ding Xue Lian
China

Yvoone Ding Xue Lian is a particularly interesting Chinese designer because she aims her work at China's internal mid-market, especially in Shanghai. She and her staff of seven other designers do all the brand designs of the Shanghai Silk Import and Export Company: men's wear, baby clothing, sportswear, women's wear, spring and autumn collections. She likes to give her designs a sense of power, often through clashing identities, such as irregular cuts and shapes. She chooses colours by feeling, looking for their strengths. In the China market, however, this can be a tricky matter. The colour red, for example, has a long history of expressing both power and luck, but it is easy to make mistakes by using red in an incorrect way.

"In China almost every mother makes her children's clothes. But my father also made clothes too, which was not so common. When I was small he made two dresses for me. That taught me that making dresses is not difficult, but fun. I devoted myself to the fashion world because I was born with an impulse to dress up. Designing is the best language I have to express that impulse.

"Garments rely on each human's existence. They can't be separated from each other any more than humans can. Nor can they be shielded from the changes in the personality and emotions of the wearer."

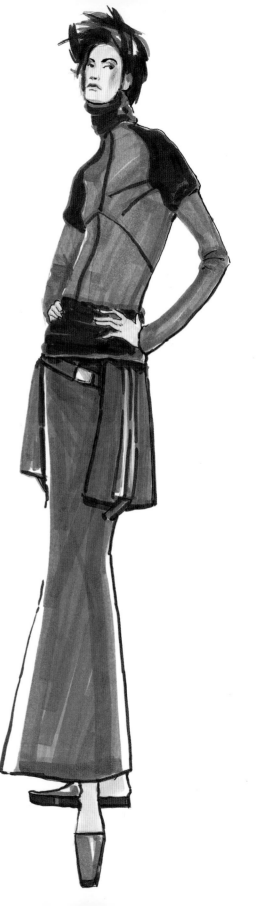

In my first three years after graduation, I had the chance to work with all kinds of clothes aimed at many different kinds of buyers. A designer working in China's brand-name market must not only understand commercial value, but also express the joys and hardships of personal feelings in their designs.

I sketch quickly while listening to music. I feel my emotions rising and falling as the musical notes turn alternately gentle and sharp. I am completely free from restraint when I sketch in the midst of music's booming reverberations.

The career of every designer must surely have stages like these, clear and leaping, rather like an aircraft flying across the sky leaving a different trail each time it passes. For me it is imperative to feel the pinnacled European church with its elegant and delicate, yet greyish, moods; to feel sunshine in the Americas, in that land's warm and bold colours; to feel the different tempos of work between merchants and artisans; to feel the sluggish musical tones in a bar and the quick and rhythmic movement of work in an office.

I must learn what attire the customers want if I am to create clothing that flies over and above the practical world of market demand. I need to open my sensitivities to the social currents behind dressmaking, get to know every facet of the customer's personal environment, adjust my thinking to theirs, get more familiar with international art developments and how these change our era. **"**

"The bird-wing image in some of my clothes is a heat-applied transfer made from my own computer design. It is my imaginary image of myself."

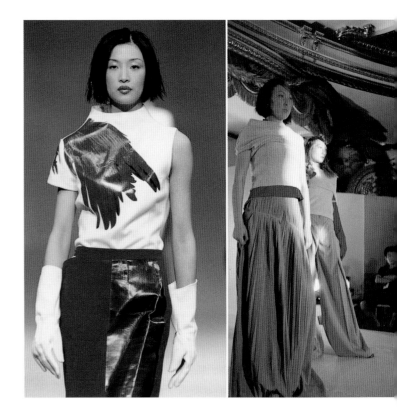

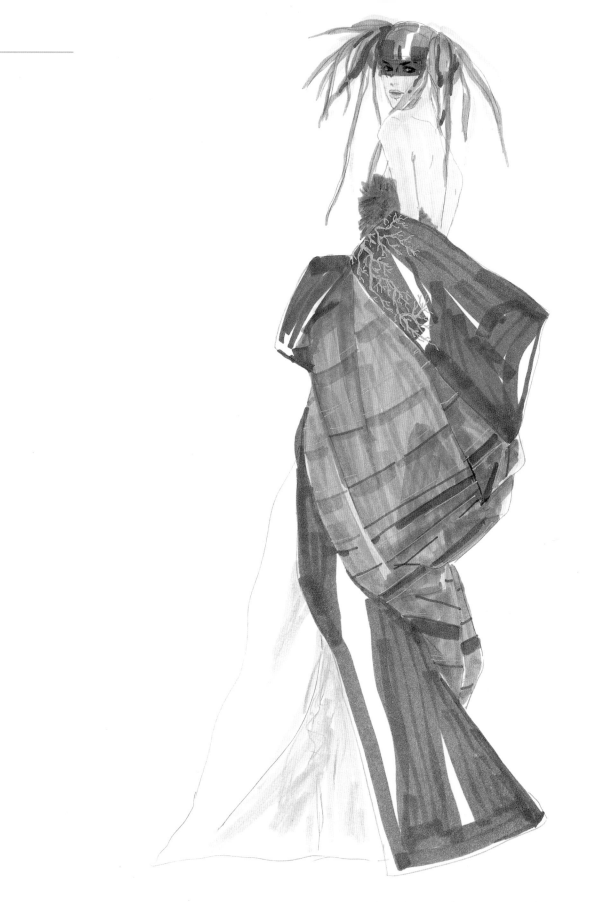

Coco Ma
China

Coco Ma believes that, in and of itself, the life of a designer is not difficult to handle. It is the business part that is hard. 'The talent of Chinese designers is good, but they need more government – as well as business – support. I started my boutique by borrowing from friends. I paid them back and now I'm on my own. But not everybody can do that.'

Then she goes on to say, 'Beauty is not in the face, it is in the heart. Beauty is when you are touched in the heart.'

"I was the youngest daughter in the family and the first known artist. Before university I liked music, dance, painting. I then studied fashion design for three years. Today I like architecture, interior design, movies, photographs, little animals – my cat is my daughter.

Some fabrics have their own life, an inner character that I can feel. When I get that feel, I choose that fabric. I try to understand its character, bring it to life with my own feelings.

"My designs are a way of looking forward. I experience with feelings – my feelings about life, about the future."

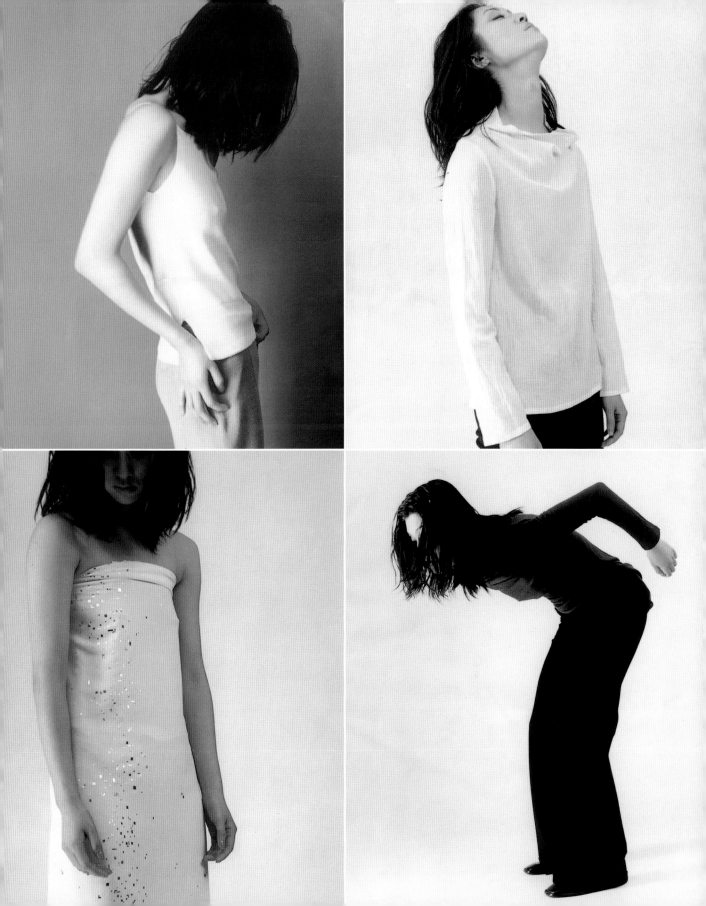

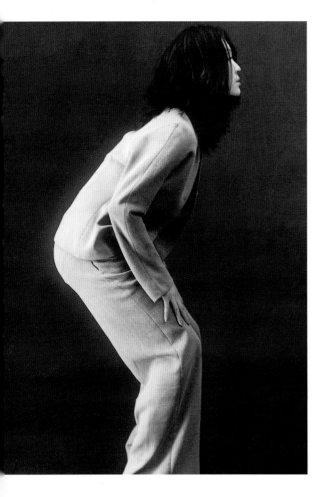

Designs come to me in two ways. Sometimes they just go 'pffft!' and there they are. Other times they must gestate. When I begin a collection, I know part of it will go into a retail store and part into a fashion boutique. The two clients are very different and I have to keep both in mind.

When I dress a woman, she should not be too glamorous. Prettiness is not in the face, it is in the heart. A woman should have simple but long-lasting clothes.

People are kind by nature. We have to nurture that. When I was in Hong Kong, walking in the street, I saw a little kitten. I talked to it and it approached me. In China, they run away. In a society, if the people are friendly and accept everything, including ideas, then their attitudes will be reflected in even the little animals.

The end of the millennium should be a time for people to take a breather, enter the new age refreshed. I hope the next millennium will be a time when different people come together, find a common space to express themselves. We need change, but we also need to keep things. **"**

"I get ideas from everywhere, but through my own lens. I love nature and draw much inspiration from it. For me, it is important that fashion should be only a small part of my life. The most important thing is to better myself. Fashion design is my way to improve myself."

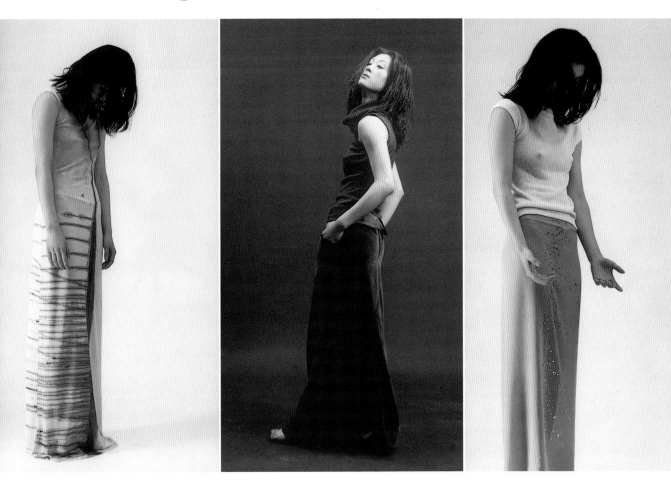

The Future

Design by Tan Yoong

What should we make of this anthill of fashion activity spread across so many locales that barely know of each other? Asian designers are so neglected by even the local press that, until now, their collective strengths and mistakes have gone unportrayed. Why does it take a Donna Karan to notice the sarong or a Jean-Paul Gaultier to do an Asian collection before the world sits up and takes notice?

Yet Asian designers' survival instincts are strong enough to have weathered an economic buffeting that, in pure financial terms, would have flattened all but the most prestigious fashion houses in the more affluent parts of the world. They have developed such an acute sensitivity to the buyer that more and more designers are bringing out a new collection every *week*.

Until designers like those discussed in this book came along, the bureaucratically anointed contemporary arts in much of Asia lived in a world of imitative make-believe. Aesthetic officialdom in Korea and Japan turned to the ballets of yesteryear and to violinists playing Brahms, while many of their artists borrowed heavily from Rauschenberg and Rothko. Thailand regilded the already encrusted dances and palaces of centuries ago. Hong Kong updated the village morality play and turned it into the Triad flick.

Self-expression in people's choice of clothing became directionless. Buyers preferred overseas names and bland tints to local hand-tailoring and richly patterned textiles. Amid all this envying of elsewhere, the most original visual artists in the region – its fashion, graphic and interior designers – were all but ignored.

But, from afar, Asians began to be nominated for the Booker Prize. A parade of Asian films won screenings at Cannes. The author Shoba De humiliated male narcissism to the collective cheers of Indian women. Singapore's Catherine Lim brought out daring novels (for Singapore, anyway) detailing the purse-lipped misery behind the Chinese wife's and bondsmaid's subservience – much to the annoyance of Lee Kuan Yew. Women's reality was expressed in truths so brutal that even the men were humbled. And then there were those legions of kids mastering the arts of the video arcade with such an intensity that few people realize that in Asia this groundswell of feelings mixed with identity has become more powerful than rock.

Clearly it wasn't all that perfect behind the facades of the governments, and the artists were beginning to say so.

It was during the 1987–1997 era of false confidence and wilful blindness that most of the fashion designers in this book evolved both

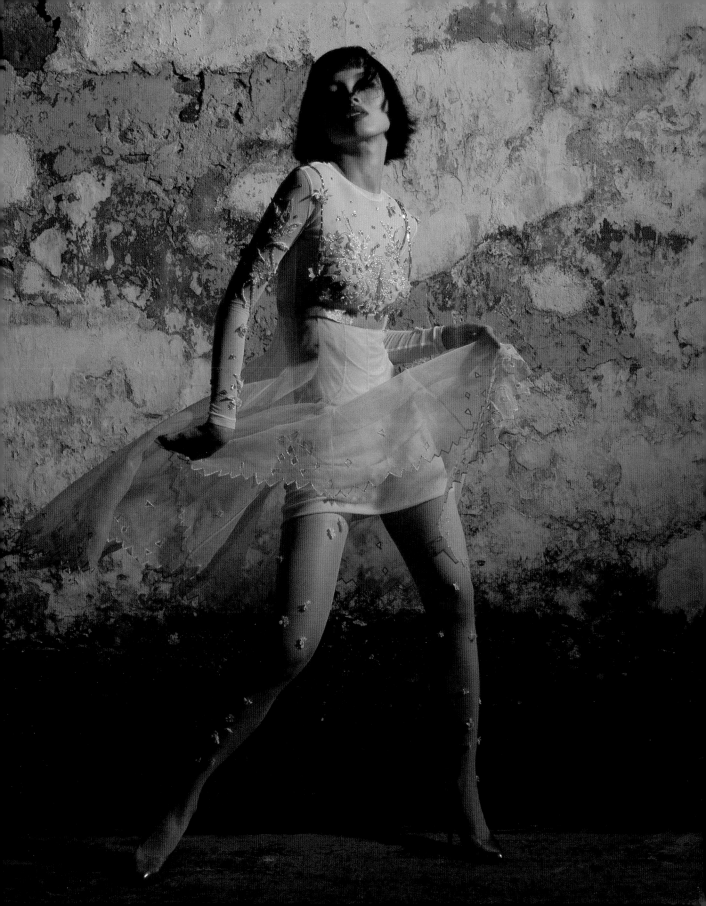

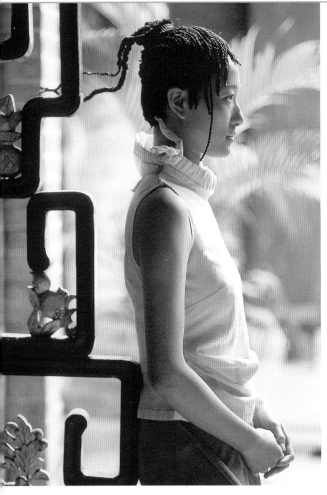

"Developing in near-isolation for so long is the best thing that could have happened to Asia's fashion designers."

their aesthetics and their markets. Which came first is hard to say. There's an endless dilemma in Asia as to whether you live it until you think it or you think it until you live it. But by whatever path, Asian fashion aesthetics have resulted in three broad trends today: modern minimalism, old wine in new bottles, and couture-à-prêt.

Two Never-Changing Trends...

Asia's fashion minimalism isn't a paring down to an irreducible minimum. Instead, it is adding to nothing to create the perfect something – just as many of the region's Missies gain shape until they're fecund, then no more until they're nearing fifty.

Old wine in new bottles is the region's most fascinating contribution. It isn't so much a vocabulary of techniques as a dictionary of histories. It is perfectly possible at certain social events in Indonesia and Thailand to squint your eyes and to be unsure as to which millennium you're in. Bernard Chandran takes us into the courts of Srivijayan Hinduism in Java and Rizalman introduces us to the palaces of the Malacca sultanates. Ghea Panggabean has already said, but it's worth repeating, 'I'm at one with every clothing maker who ever was.'

Old wine in new bottles is perhaps the most influential idea to have emerged from the formative decade – the 1980s – of the Asian fashion identity. It is not like Western retro, looking back on bygone success. Rather, it projects the best of the past on to the tastes of the present. Sometimes this results in a direct quotation, such as a cheongsam cut from completely unadorned fabric. The absence of embroidery and ornament on a garment so traditionally associated with a profusion of such decoration can be startling at first; it gives the cheongsam an entirely new identity. Other times, the old wine is a timeless historical image such as the Chinese dragon or Malay *awang larat* (unending cloud) decorative theme, and the new bottle is a dress whose simplicity of shape is so popular today.

... And One Ever-Changing Trend

Couture-à-prêt (literally made-to-order ready-to-wear) is the logical outcome of both of the above. Its inventors and chief practitioners are Peter Teo in Singapore and Kevin Yeung in Hong Kong, although many of the others have dabbled with it in some way.

The concept behind couture-à-prêt is that, while refurbishing the historical ideas of old wine in new bottles is appropriate for weddings and social functions, few of the modern generation wear such garments at five-star hotels and business meetings. Working women choose modern minimalism for office hours. However, they opt not for the traditional tailoring of Asia's past, but for imported ready-to-wear with an impressive label – or at least whenever they can afford to. Their big dilemma is how to look chic and with-it the rest of the time.

Their needs have had a strong effect on the thinking of many Asian designers. As clothing manufacturers in an era when the trend life of the average mass-market consumer item is between a few weeks and a few months, they face the question of how to design a line that changes quickly enough for every buyer to feel they're wearing a garment that is virtually unique to them.

Couture-à-prêt originated as a designer response to the above. It has now become a fashion style all of its own. It links the region's typically tiny production shops with the instant feedback that department stores can provide from their barcoded cash registers. In sum, it means making very quick changes to a design theme, based upon what buyers have chosen from Thursday through to Saturday. By Saturday night, the stores know what has sold. By Sunday morning, the designers know what has worked. By Monday morning, they are devising a dozen variations based on last week's successes. By Tuesday morning, the revisions are at the juki machines. By Wednesday afternoon, the tiny production runs – eight to a dozen garments of a dozen designs in three sizes – are complete. By Thursday morning, they are on display, ready for the next buying week. It is as close to made-to-order as ready-to-wear can be. (It is also a system that would not work very well outside the milieu of Asia's narrow range of body shapes.)

Couture-à-prêt has an important future in Asia, since Asia isn't merely billions of people, it is also thousands of market niches.

Today's couture-à-prêt buyers see their future very differently compared to a few short years ago. Instead of a blossoming of confidence and affluence, they anticipate the gloomy inheritance tax of the older generation's profligacy. They realize their leaders have endangered Asia's economic future with political styles based on pomp before performance and business styles based on conspicuous construction.

Couture-à-prêt is the kind of homegrown solution that tends to emerge in times like these. It is a meaningful response to the problem of so few Asian small business owners being adept at adding value to goods where the need is greatest: satisfying customers.

A New and Different Fashion Buyer

Today's fresh-faced MBA graduates are back from Princeton or Cambridge. They are talking service industry where their fathers talked manufacturing. They are talking about local customers in the way their fathers talked about overseas consumers. They are talking about entrepreneurialism where their fathers talked about corporatism. It is inevitable that their sense of hope fighting history will develop its own unique aesthetic tastes. Ironically, had those MBA graduates studied their home markets, they would have seen the solution underway long ago, in the couture-à-prêt approach of their own tiny fashion communities.

Of all the fashion ideas we have seen in this book, the one most attuned to the consumer-market realities of today is couture-à-prêt. True, the magnificences of the past are worth retaining and old wine in new bottles will endure at least until the last of today's dowagers have gone, and perhaps longer among those of their daughters who can't bear to throw away all those memories. But these daughters also see television antennae in the countryside instead of the fine weavings and embroidery of the past. Many of Asia's resource pool of village craftsmen and women are letting commercial establishments take over the roles they used to fulfil, while they ease the days away watching the soaps.

Modern minimalism, too, will stay. Bodies are bodies and sex is sex, and the age eighteen to twenty-five women's magazines still write as if nothing else matters.

Right now, the old has gone and the new hasn't yet arrived. Young Asians are grasping for, or holding on to, any identity that works. The economic rise of the Asian Tigers came in like a king and left like a stallholder. Now the fashion designers are picking up the pieces of today and, in their own special way, defining what kind of tomorrow can be made from the mistakes of yesterday.

Note: Due to the complexities of first and family names in Asia, the following list has been alphabetized by the name order used in the respective countries.

Sharifah Meheran Barakbah
Barakaff
I-23, First Floor
Star Hill Shopping Centre
Jalan Bukit Bintang
55100 Kuala Lumpur
Malaysia
Tel: 603 243-4534
Mobile: 010 227-9854

Didi Budiardjo
Jalan Bendi Besar #20
Jakarta Selatan
Indonesia
Tel: 6221 723-9540
Fax: 6221 725-0210

Carmanita
Jalan Wijaya Timur Raya #99
Jakarta 12170
Indonesia
Tel/Fax: 6221 739-7380

Allan Chai
Allan Chai Fashion Design
Peninsula Plaza
111 North Bridge Road #05-56/58
Singapore 0617
Tel/Fax: 65 338-4330

William Chan
Menage à Toi
12FL, New York House
60 Connaught Road, Central
Hong Kong
Tel: 852 2722-1510
Fax: 852 2722-5506

Bernard Chandran
Box 68
2nd Floor
Kuala Lumpur Plaza
Bukit Bintang
55100 Kuala Lumpur
Malaysia
Mobile: 012 283-6601
        010 229-1320
Fax: 603 254-0534

Jamei Chen
1F, No. 23, Lane 219
Fu Hsing South Road, Section 1
Taipei
Taiwan, RoC
Tel: 886-2 2751-7989
Fax: 886-2 2741-2752

Shiatzy Chen
Shiatzy International Co., Ltd
49-1, Chung Shan North Road,
Section 2
Taipei 10419
Taiwan, RoC
Tel: 886-2 2542-5506
Fax: 886-2 2561-5601

Bonita Cheung
Tassels Couture
9th Floor
California Entertainment Building
34–36 D'Aguilar Street, Central
Hong Kong
Tel: 852 2868-2820
Mobile: 852 9435-1000
Fax: 852 2868-1130
E-mail: tassels@vol.net

Lu Lu Cheung
Rolls Group Ltd
3/F, Block A, Chung Mei Centre
15 Hing Yip Street
Kwun Tong, Kowloon
Hong Kong
Tel: 852 2793-0830
Fax: 852 2342-6308
E-mail: rollsgrp@netvigator.com

Yvoone Ding Xue Lian
Shanghai Silk Imp. & Exp. Co., Ltd,
O.I.C.
16F, 1666–1686 Si Chuan Road (N)
Global New Times Plaza
Shanghai 200080
China
Tel: 86-21 6357-2288/2052
Fax: 86-21 6393-9214
E-mail: DCG@SHSILK.COM.CN

**Stephane Dou and
Changlee Yugin**
Stephane Dou International Co., Ltd
3F, No. 34-2, Lane 391, Section 3
Ho-Ping East Road
Taipei
Taiwan, RoC
Tel: 886-2 2378-3629
Fax: 886-2 2735-2791

Ronald Gaghana
Jalan Villa Sawo Kav 25
Cipete Utara
Kebayoran Baru
Jakarta Selatan 12150
Indonesia
Tel: 6221 724-8086
Fax: 6221 723-2786

Cesar Gaupo
Cesar Gaupo, Inc.
#3 First Street
Villamar Compound
Tambo, Parañaque
Metro Manila
The Philippines
Tel: 632 831-6634
Fax: 632 551-3368

Sebastian Gunawan
Harmoni Plaza
Jalan Suryopranoto #2
Block K #1
Jakarta Selatan 10130
Indonesia
Tel: 6221 384-7790
Fax: 6221 630-3433

Sophie Hong
Sophie Hong Fashion
20, Lane 7
Yung Kang Street
Taipei
Taiwan, RoC
Tel: 886-2 2351-6469
Fax: 886-2 2517-8173
E-mail: Pigeonzi@ms21.hinet.net

Ika
Butoni Ltd
20 Hillwood Road
8/F Kam Hing Building
Tsimshatsui, Kowloon
Hong Kong
Tel: 852 2724-1818
Fax: 852 2739-5597
E-mail: butoni@hkstar.com

Bill Keith
78A Jalan Alor
off Changkat Bukit Bintang
50200 Kuala Lumpur
Malaysia
Tel/Fax: 603 242-6646
Mobile: 018 830-3573

Ann Kelly *see* **Wykidd Song**

Peter Lau
XCVIII Limited
Shop 1, LG/F
65 Kimberley Road
Tsimshatsui, Kowloon
Hong Kong
Mobile: 852 9641-1702
Fax: 852 2367-9979
E-mail: xcviiico@super.net

Lee Kuann-I
Lee Kuann-I Design Co., Ltd
Pa-Teh Road 2nd
Section No. 227
3F Taipei
Taiwan, RoC
Tel: 886-2 2711-8082
Fax: 886-2 2714-8635

Leung Thong Ping
Mayfair Designs
Lot FF-008 (Tingkat 1)
Bukit Bintang Plaza
Jalan Bukit Bintang
55100 Kuala Lumpur
Malaysia
Tel/Fax: 603 242-7441

Celia Loe
First Stop Private Ltd
5 Pereira Road
#05-03 Asiawide Industrial Building
Singapore 368025
Tel: 65 287-8284
Fax: 65 281-0090

Coco Ma
Mixmind Art & Design Studio
Room C3, 6/F No. 1 Door
Golden Bridge Building
No. 93, SiYou New Road
WuYang New City
Guangzhou
China
Tel/Fax: 86-20 8738-1168/8263
E-mail: exception@163.net

Walter Ma
Front First Ltd
Unit 11, 8/F, Tower 1
Harbour Centre
1 Hok Cheung Street
Hung Hom, Kowloon
Hong Kong
Tel: 852 2764-8673/8674/
8675/8676
Fax: 852 2774-6253
E-mail: gee@netvigator.com
http://www.sme-cma.org.hk/
compro/walterma

Nagara
28 Ladpraord
Soi 199
Bangkok 10310
Thailand
Tel: 662 514-3130
Fax: 662 530-2210
E-mail: nagara@ksc.th.com

Cynthia Ng Meng Sim
Block 14, #12-957
Upper Boon Keng Road
Singapore 380014
Tel: 65 745-8619
Mobile: 65 9223-7136
E-mail: ncwmsg@pacific.net.sg

Carven Ong
10 First Floor
Kan Cho Hong
Jalan Panggong
50000 Kuala Lumpur
Malaysia
Tel: 603 201-3391
Fax: 603 238-7128

Ghea Panggabean
Ghea Fashion Studio
Pusat Pertokoan
Permata Hijau Blok D–B/18
Jakarta Selatan 12210
Indonesia
Tel: 6221 533-1972
Fax: 6221 549-3249

Sahasab Pinprachasan
Preti Boutique
20/6 Soi Prompong
Sukhumvit 39
Bangkok 10110
Thailand
Tel: 662 258-3422
Fax: 662 261-6562

House of Prajudi
Mr Ari Saputra
Jalan Hang Lekir VI/5
Kebayoran Baru
Jakarta Selatan 12120
Indonesia
Tel: 6221 724-3680
Fax: 6221 739-8668

Rizalman
A Scent of Lace
Lot 012B, 2nd Floor
Bukit Bintang Plaza
55100 Kuala Lumpur
Malaysia
Tel: 603 243-0608
Mobile: 010-227-7159

Lily Salim
Parti Salim Garmindo Indah
Jalan Praja F7
Kebayoran Lama
Jakarta 12240
Indonesia
Tel: 6221 724-8092
Fax: 6221 739-8413

Edmund Ser
49 Jalan 3/23A
Danau Kota
off Jalan Genting Kelang
Setapak
53300 Kuala Lumpur
Malaysia
Tel: 603 245-9201/9202/9203
9204/9205/9206
Fax: 603 411-7228

Wykidd Song and Ann Kelly
Song & Kelly
27-A Mosque Street
Singapore 059505
Tel: 65 323-4035
Fax: 65 323-0296

Inno Sotto
Inno Sotto Luxe Wear
2021 M.H. Del Pilar
South Syquia
Malate
1004 Manila
The Philippines
Tel: 632 524-9782/632 521-8195/
632 524-7656 x208
Fax: 632 522-3591

William Tang
William Tang Co., Ltd
99 Hang Tau Tsuen
Ping Shan, New Territories
Hong Kong
Tel: 852 2545-5526
Fax: 852 2815-7384

Esther Tay
Paul Chua
Estabelle Fashions Private Ltd
Block 1001
Jalan Bukit Merah #04-11/12
Redhill Industrial Estate
Singapore 159455
Tel: 65 375-8033
Fax: 65 272-3421

Peter Teo
Project Shop/Blood Brothers
Fashion Mart
Building B/1C, 10th Floor 7M
60B Martin Road
Singapore 239065
Tel: 65 8363-7161
E-mail: bloodbrs@pacific.net.sg

Patis Tesoro
169 Wilson Street
San Juan 1500
Metro Manila
The Philippines
Tel: 632 726-5058/5059
Fax: 632 724-6203
E-mail: patis@katutubo.org
titot@epic.net

Kevin Tsao Yao-Wen
Block 2, Pandan Valley #03-203
Singapore 597626
Tel: 65 467-1675
Mobile: 65 9794-6707

Rowena U
GeRoyle Fashion Industries Ltd
901-3 Conic Investment Building
13 Hok Yuen Street
Hung Hom, Kowloon
Hong Kong
Tel: 852 2954-1331
Fax: 852 2356-7328

Pacino Wan
She & He Ltd
Block D, 24/F
Jing Ho Industrial Building
78–84 Wang Lung Street
Tsuen Wan, New Territories
Kowloon, Hong Kong
Tel: 852 2408-2151
Fax: 852 2409-118

Biyan Wanaatmadja
Plaza Senayan
2nd Floor
Jakarta Selatan
Indonesia
Tel: 6221 724-8086
Fax: 6221 723-2786

Benny Yeung
Ben Yeung Ltd
8/F, Canton House
54-56 Queen's Road, Central
Hong Kong
Tel: 852 2523-1319
Fax: 852 2522-2751

Kevin Yeung
Gobelins Company
Unit L, 9/F, Kaiser Estate
Second Phase
51 Man Yue Street
Hung Hom, Kowloon
Hong Kong
Tel: 852 2764-2378
Fax: 852 2363-7500

Tan Yoong
Tan Yoong Creations Private Ltd
304 Orchard Road #02-50
Lucky Plaza
Singapore 238863
Tel: 65 734-3783
65 235-2113
Fax: 65 732-8870
E-mail: tanyoong@singnet.com.sg
www.tanyoong.com

Changlee Yugin *see* **Stephane Dou**

Acknowledgments

Gazing back over the many people who helped this book come into being is like looking over your flower garden in spring: such a joy to behold, and so many memories to retain!

In Jakarta, Yenny Tan of the Indonesian Fashion Design Council arranged for all the interviews with the designers and, in addition, a custom photo shoot of the work of most of the Indonesians in this book. She worked under the guidance of Dipl. Des. Sjamsidar Isa, President of the IFDC. Mr Olly Ganjar Santosa, consultant to the IFDC, hosted several interview sessions and gave much useful background information about the historical development of the Jakarta fashion community. The unseen presence of Susan Budihardjo and her eponymously named prestigious fashion school was like a majestic eminence behind the scrim, so important was her influence on the evolution of contemporary fashion as an art form rather than a purely commercial enterprise in Indonesia.

In Singapore, Wendy Lam, Trade Officer for the Lifestyle Business Section of Singapore's Trade Development Board (http://www.tdb.gov.sg) arranged for the photographs of the work of Cynthia Ng Meng Sim, Peter Teo and Kevin Tsao Yao-Wen. Allan Koh of D&A Management Consultants, Private Ltd gave considerable time and insight into the past development and future direction of Singapore's fashion identity. Esther Tay and her husband Paul Chua not only devoted much time and energy to the success of the project, but are also ambulatory experts on the best restaurants in Singapore! Ross Chng of Allan Chai Fashion Design provided Allan Chai's pictures. Tan Yoong is the sole owner and retains the exclusive copyright to the images published on a one-off basis in this book.

The images of the work of Malaysian designers Sharifah Barakbah, Bill Keith, Carven Ong, Rizalman and Edmund Ser were provided courtesy of the generous assistance of Sunitha Chhabra and Margaret Sebastian of *Her World* magazine in Kuala Lumpur. They are reproduced by the permission of the Berita Publishing, Sdn. Bhd, Malaysia. Sunitha Chhabra also coordinated and styled the photo shoots, and the photographers were Ikram Ismail, Shahrul Azher Shahbudin, and Haji Saleh Osman. Bernard Chandran provided his own images, which have been reproduced with his permission.

Early research about the fashion community in Thailand was furthered by valuable web site referrals from Supaporn Vathanaprida (suvathan@kcls.org). Much insight and advice was given by Mr B. Magee of Qesat Ltd (asiaexpat@hotmail.com), a commercial firm doing business with Thai exporters. His information was amplified by Pam Sreshthaputra Siam Thida Co., Ltd in Hong Kong. Once in Bangkok, Khun Napapan of the International Affairs Department at Chulalongkorn University was a fount of knowledge and helpful connections; indeed, she was largely responsible for locating the actual addresses of the Thai designers. Eric Booth, Marketing Manager of the Jim Thompson Thai Silk Co., Ltd arranged for the interview with Thailand's foremost silk designer, Nagara. Sahasab Pinprachasan was initially discovered at the 1999 Hong Kong Fashion Week and located via the assistance of the Office of Product Development and Design for Export of Thai Silk. Finally, Vithivas Khongkhakul, of the Duang Prateep Foundation, gave numerous insights into the hidden world of the Thai economic and social picture, especially about how liberating oneself via the arts is a notable success among the youngest and the poorest levels of Thai society.

Inno Sotto coordinated the site visit to Manila, with additional supporting information and insight from Liza Ilarde, Fashion and Beauty Editor of *Mega* magazine in Manila. All of Cesar Gaupo's photographs were taken by Raymon Isaac of the Philippines. Patis Tesoro's photographs were taken by Mr Neal Oshima.

The Taiwan Textiles Federation is far and away the

most impressive garment industry association in Asia and a perfect example of why Taiwan does so well despite the economic buffeting elsewhere in Asia. The TTF helps the country's textiles and fashion industries work together to develop sophisticated design and marketing organizations in their own enterprises. The TTF also represents both communities at trade shows and conventions. All my visits to and in Taiwan were arranged with the very generous assistance of Mr Justin Huang, Director of the Textile & Fashion Design Centre at the TTF (http://www.chinainc.com/categories/textile-main.htm). Josephine Lin of the TTF Design Promotion Department arranged the visits with the designers represented in this book. Michelle Chiang of the Design Development Section provided a lucid and impressive presentation of the TTF's sophisticated liaison services between Taiwanese fabric makers, fashion designers, and exporters. Once out the doors of the TTF, Feeling Chen and Sabrina Chen (accompanied by baby-to-be!) of the Design Promotion Section remained cool and collected guides-cum-taxi-hailers despite the tight schedule and many madcap rides all over Taipei – and even managed to throw in visits to a few of Taipei's tourist attractions as well!

At the individual designer level, Françoise Zylerberg of Moishe Ltd was very helpful in unveiling the ideas hidden beneath the surface of Sophie Hong's design – not to mention her introductions at the many little arts cafés tucked away in hard-to-find quarters of the city. Shiatzy Chen was a delightful fount of ideas and graciousness – and knew how to find the best shark's fin soup in Taipei! Stephane Dou and Changlee Yugin's designs were photographed by Terence Huang, Taipei.

Thanks, too, to Jenny Yi Chen, Fashion Editor of *Bazaar*, Taipei; Ing-Jiuan Wang, Reporter for *The Liberty Times*, Taipei; Amber Chen, Executive Editor for *Taiwan Vogue*; Diane Ying, Editor/Publisher of *CommonWealth*, Taipei; and Lena Yang, Editor-in-Chief of *Elle* in Taipei. All of these gave their own perceptions of Taipei's fashion world. I don't know who paid for the dinner, but many *many* thanks!

And still in Taiwan, many thanks to Chinese Fancy Leather Industry Co., Ltd, Forward Textile Co., Ltd, Lee Fang Enterprise Co., Merryson Corporation, Tung Zong Textile Co., Ltd and Yu Yuang Textile Co., Ltd.

The Hong Kong Fashion Designers Association and Hong Kong Trade Development Council (who can be contacted at hktdc@tdc.org.hk; http://www.tdc.org.hk) are responsible for the success of Hong Kong's representation in this book. Special thanks to Porcia Leung of the HKTDC's public relations coordinator, Occasions/PR Network, who largely arranged the visit, with further help from Agnes Chan, the HKTDC's Manager of Fashion Promotion. Assistance in meeting specific designers came from Angy Shum and William Chan's aide-in-chief (and aspiring model) Lillian Ho.

Ms Song Wenwen of the China Fashion Designers Association in Beijing was instrumental in solving the intractable communications and delivery problems inherent in dealing with a fashion community spread over a vast country. For further information about China's design community, she may be contacted at ray.zhou@263.net and zhangtingwin@263.net.

Beyond these individuals, I too must thank Jamie Camplin at Thames & Hudson for his imperturbable patience during those many times when the parts of this book seemed to be flying in every direction except towards a manuscript binder. Literary agent Barbara Braun in New York kept her finger on the pulse of production, fluttery at times though that pulse was. Once the flutters became a pulse, the Thames & Hudson team and the book's designer, Avril Broadley, waved magic wands over everything to produce the finery you see now.

And most and thus last, to my dearest friend, Diane Freburg in California, who kept the fires of faith flickering during those long months with no e-mails, no pictures, and not much left in the budget.